This Coloring Book Belongs to

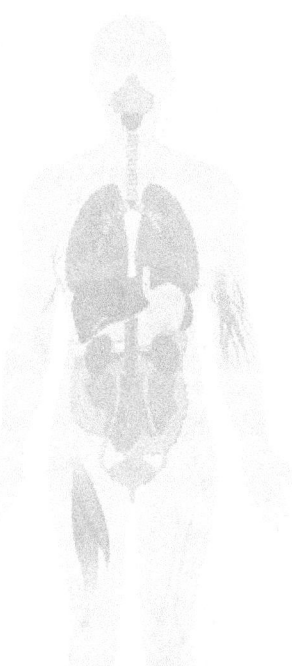

Copyright © Tfatef Toura

All rights reserved. No parts of this publication may be reproduced, distributed, or transmitted in any form, or by any means, including photocopying, recording or other electronic or mechanical methods, without prior written permission from the publisher.

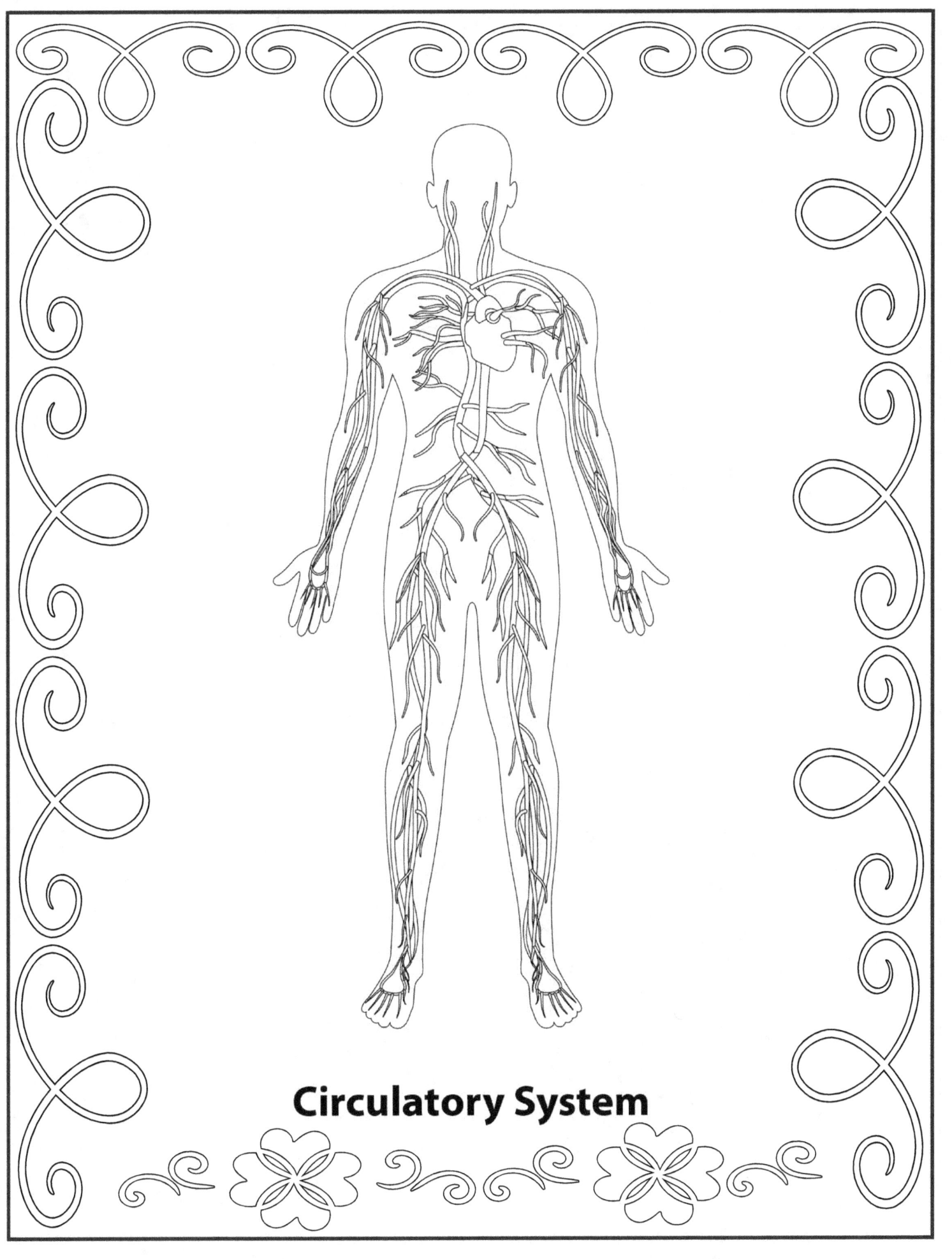

Circulatory System

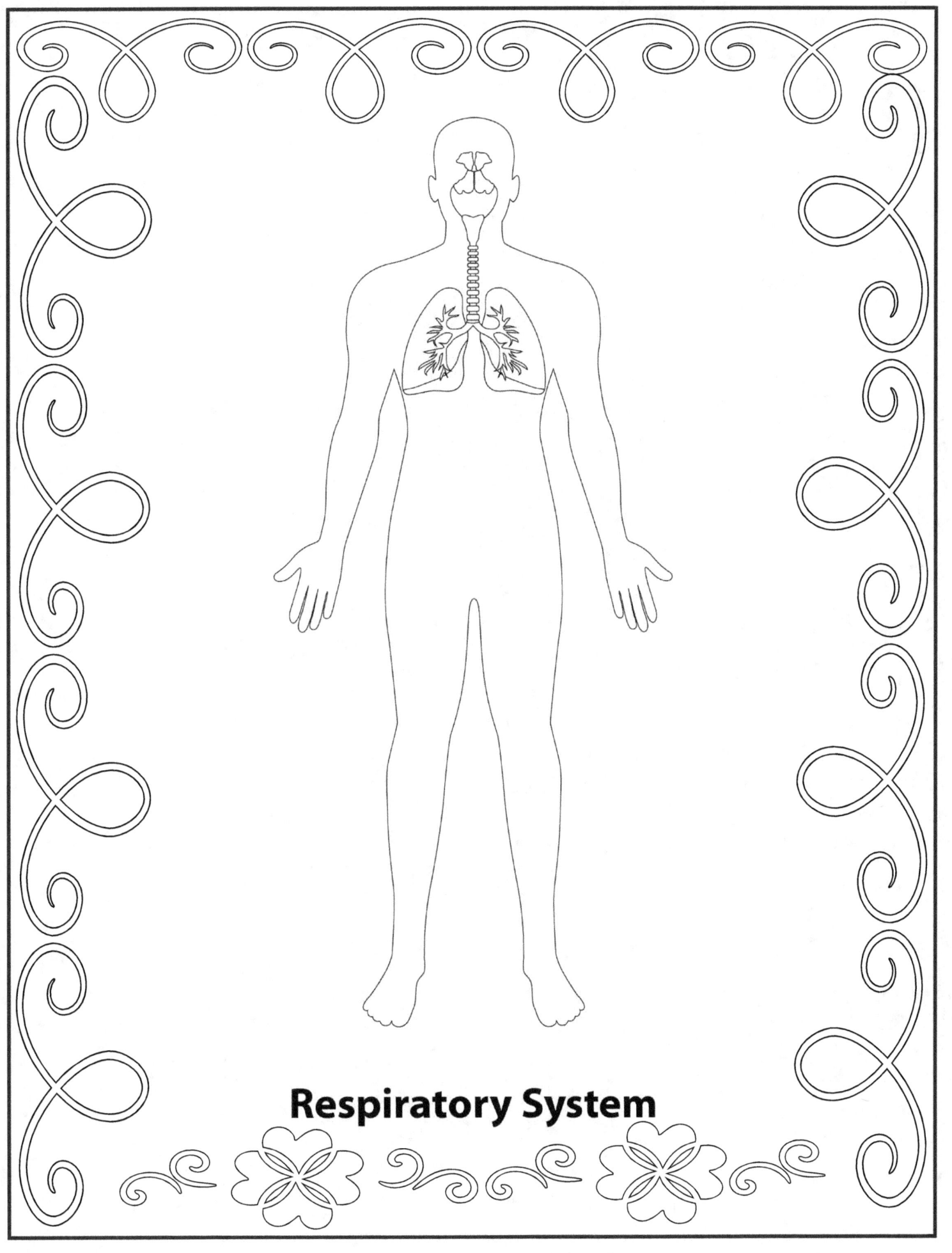

Respiratory System

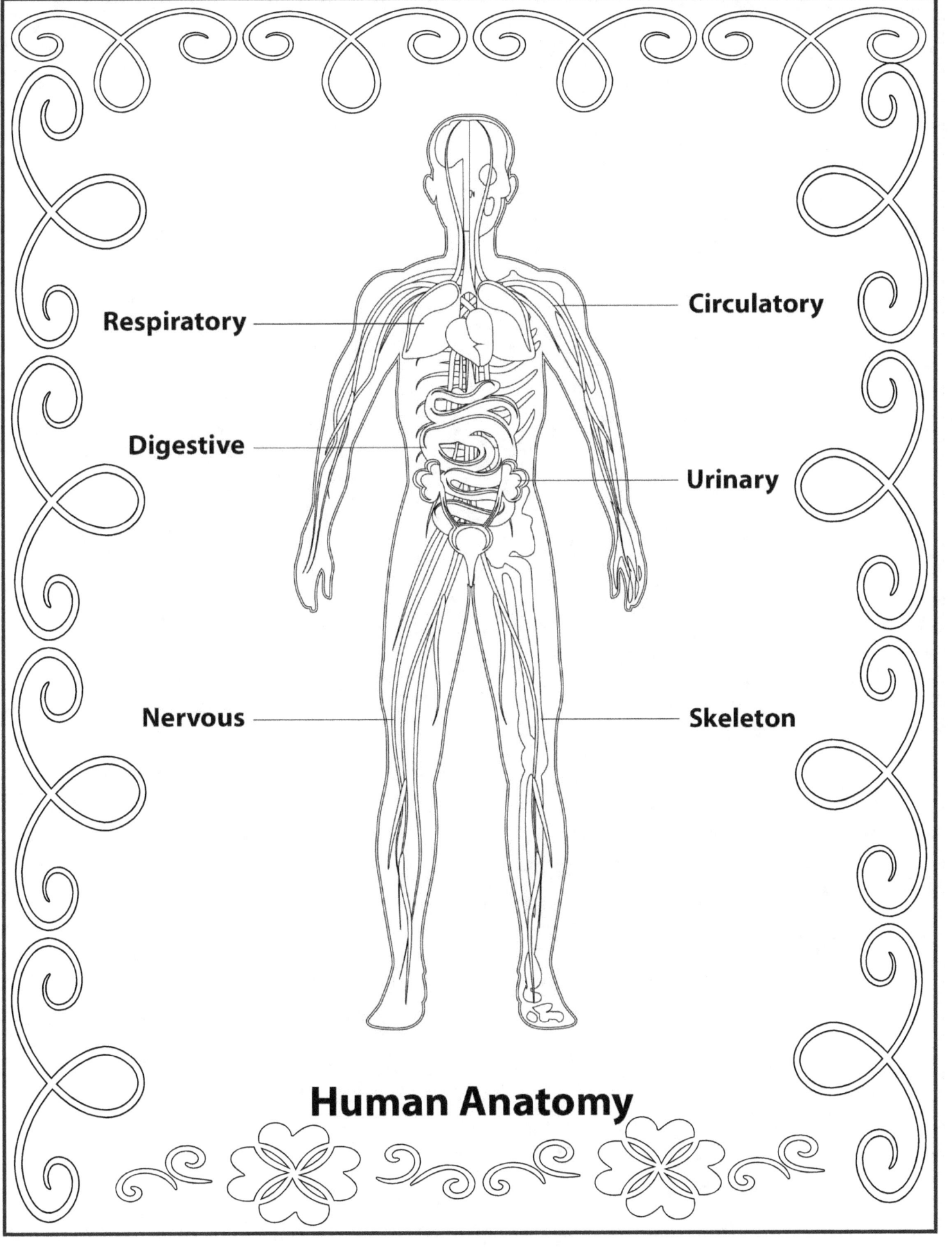

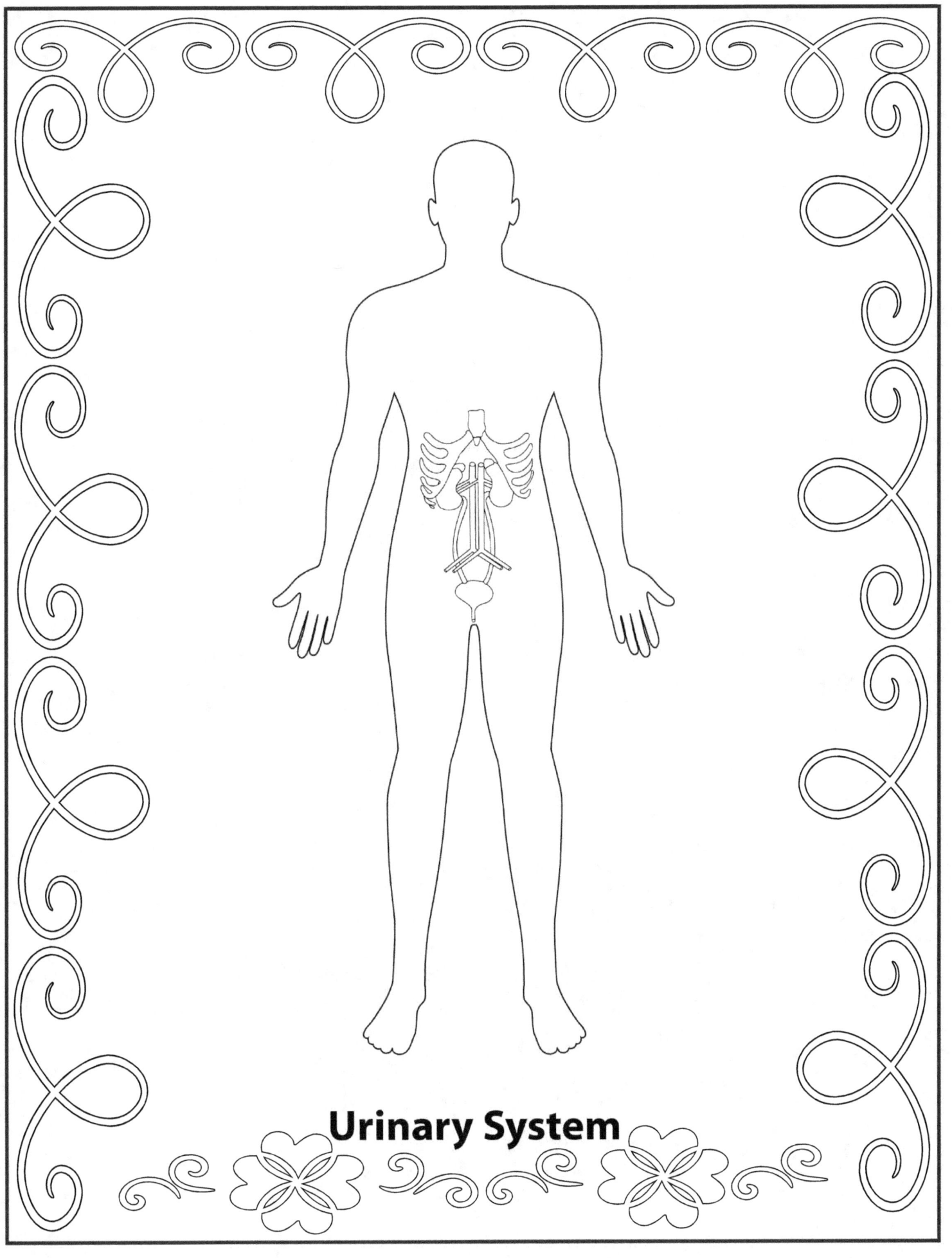

Urinary System

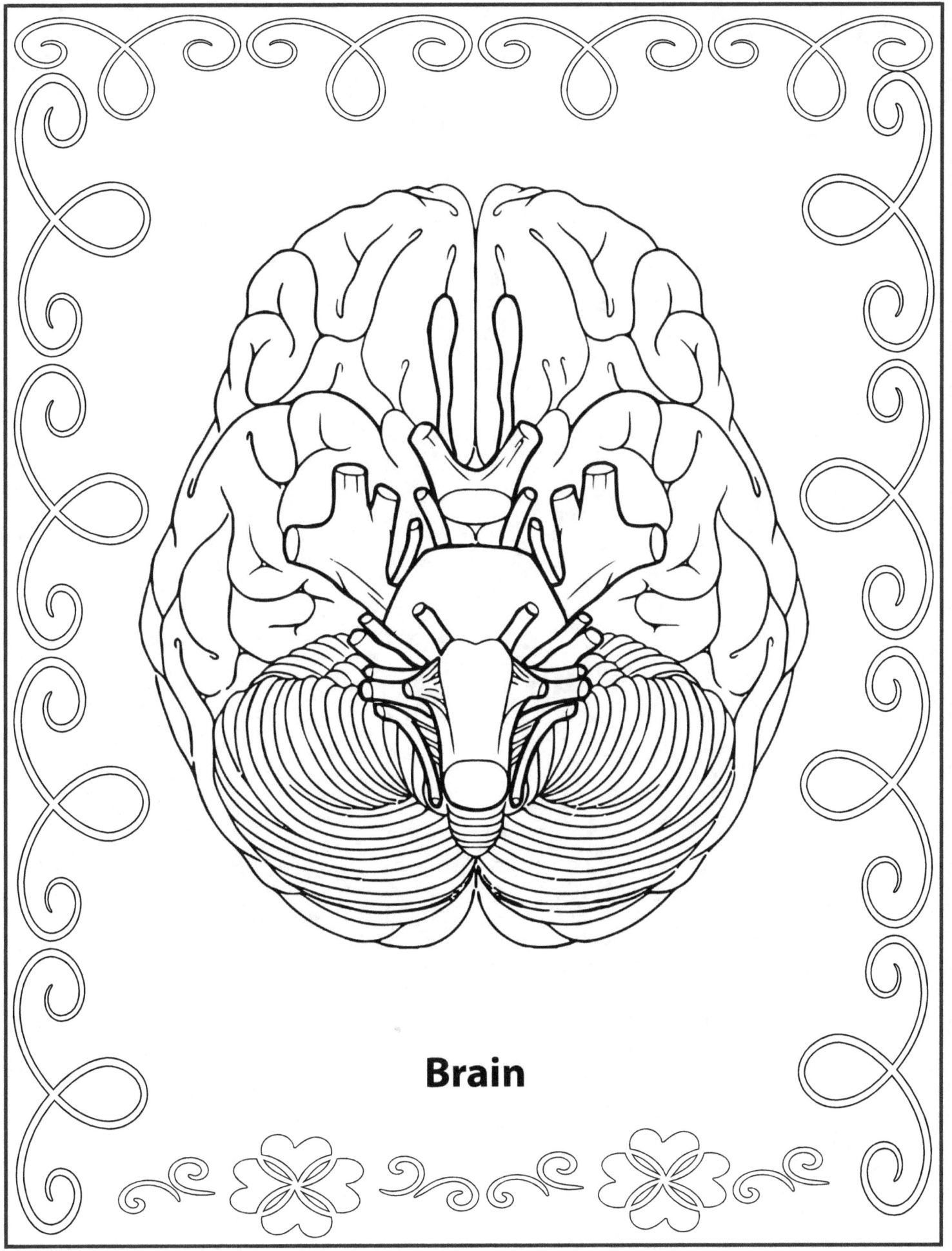

Brain

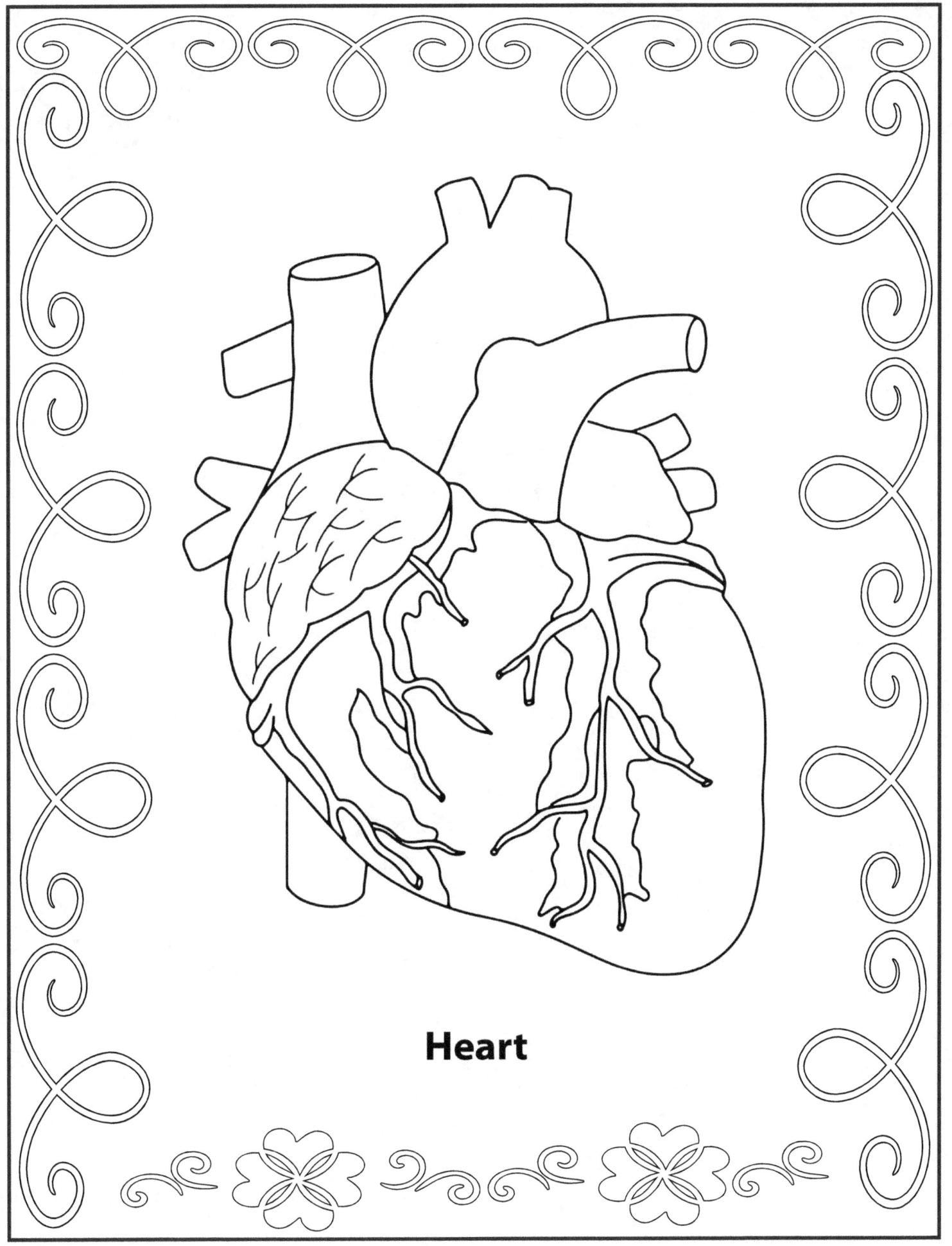
Heart

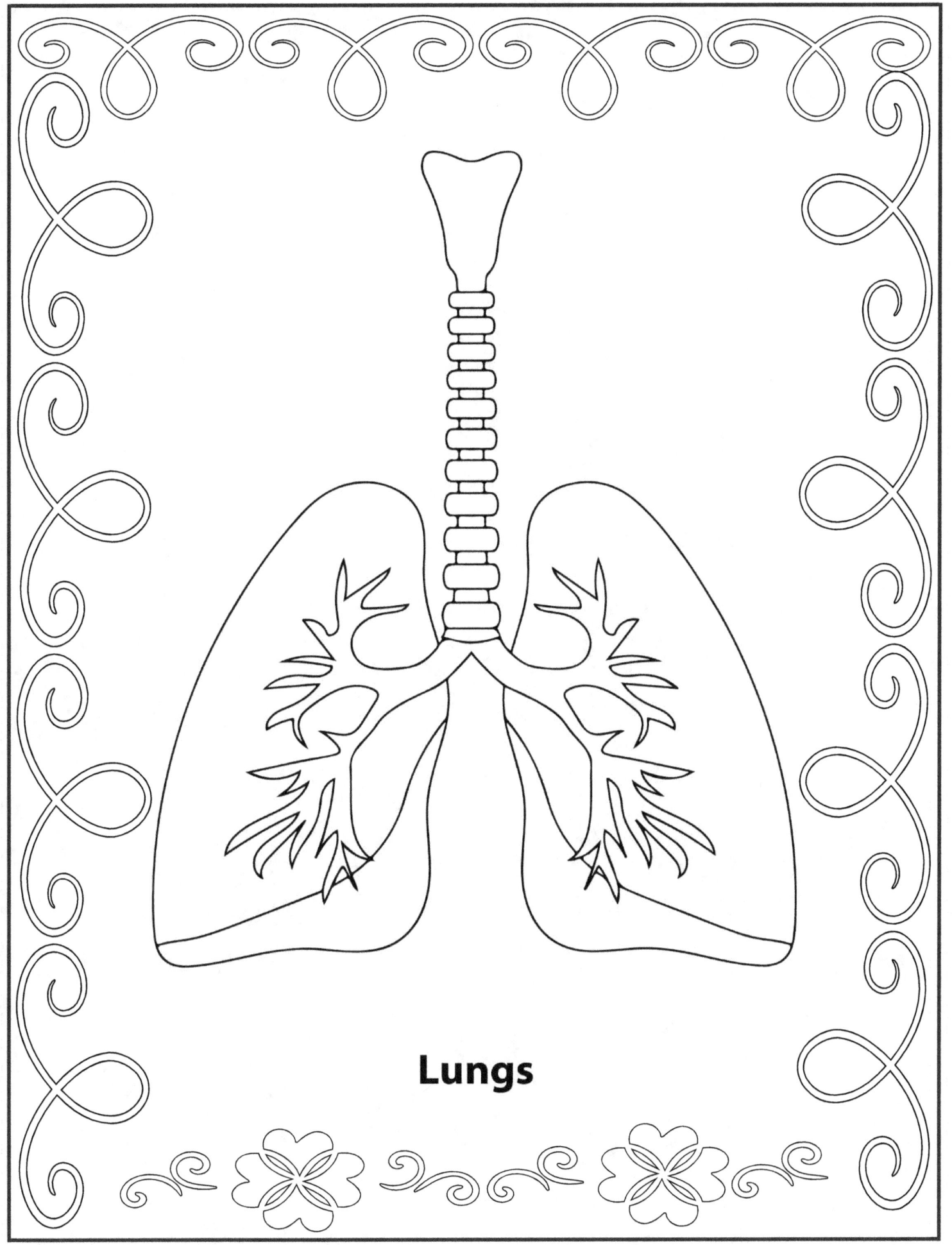

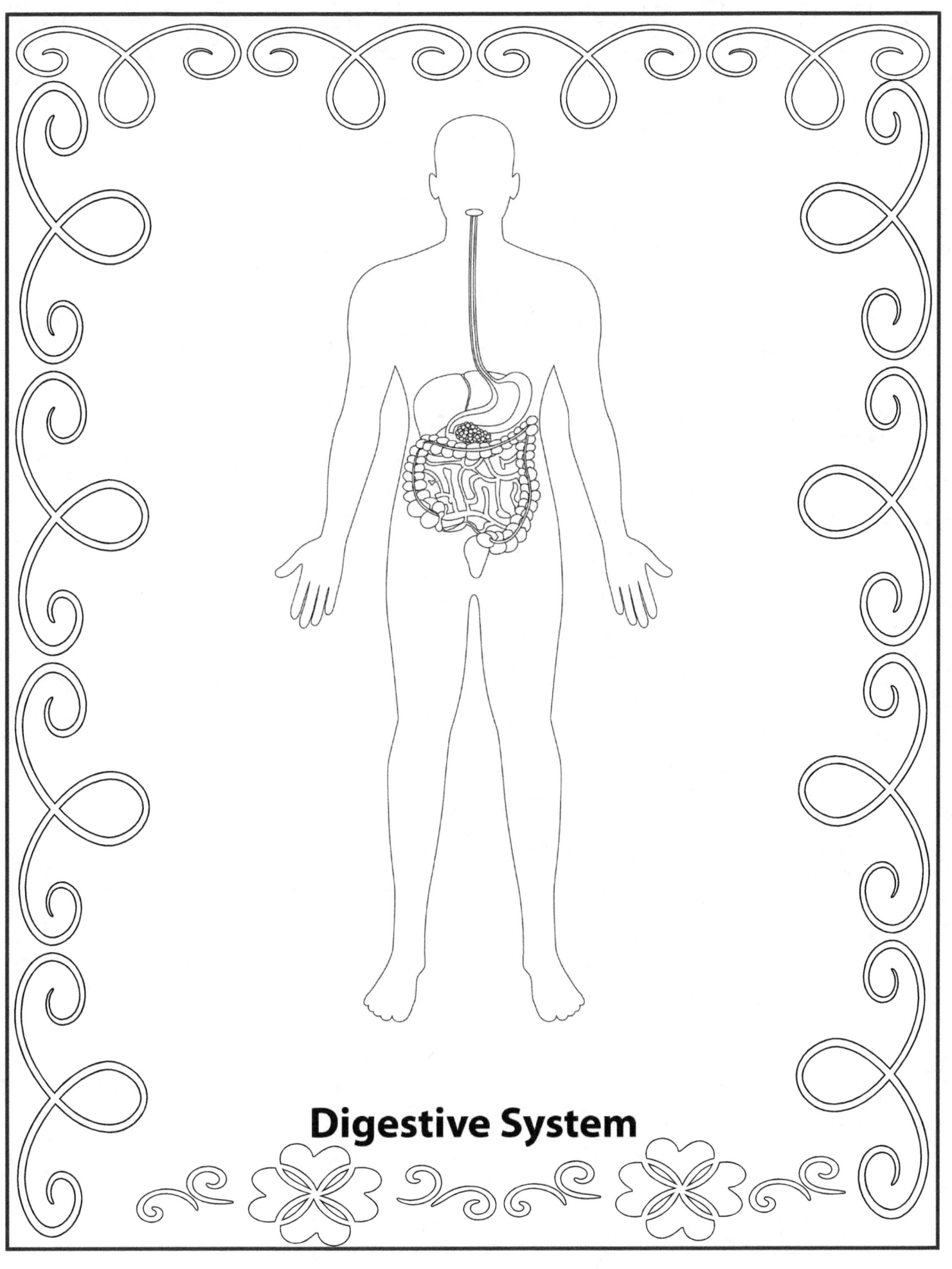

Digestive System

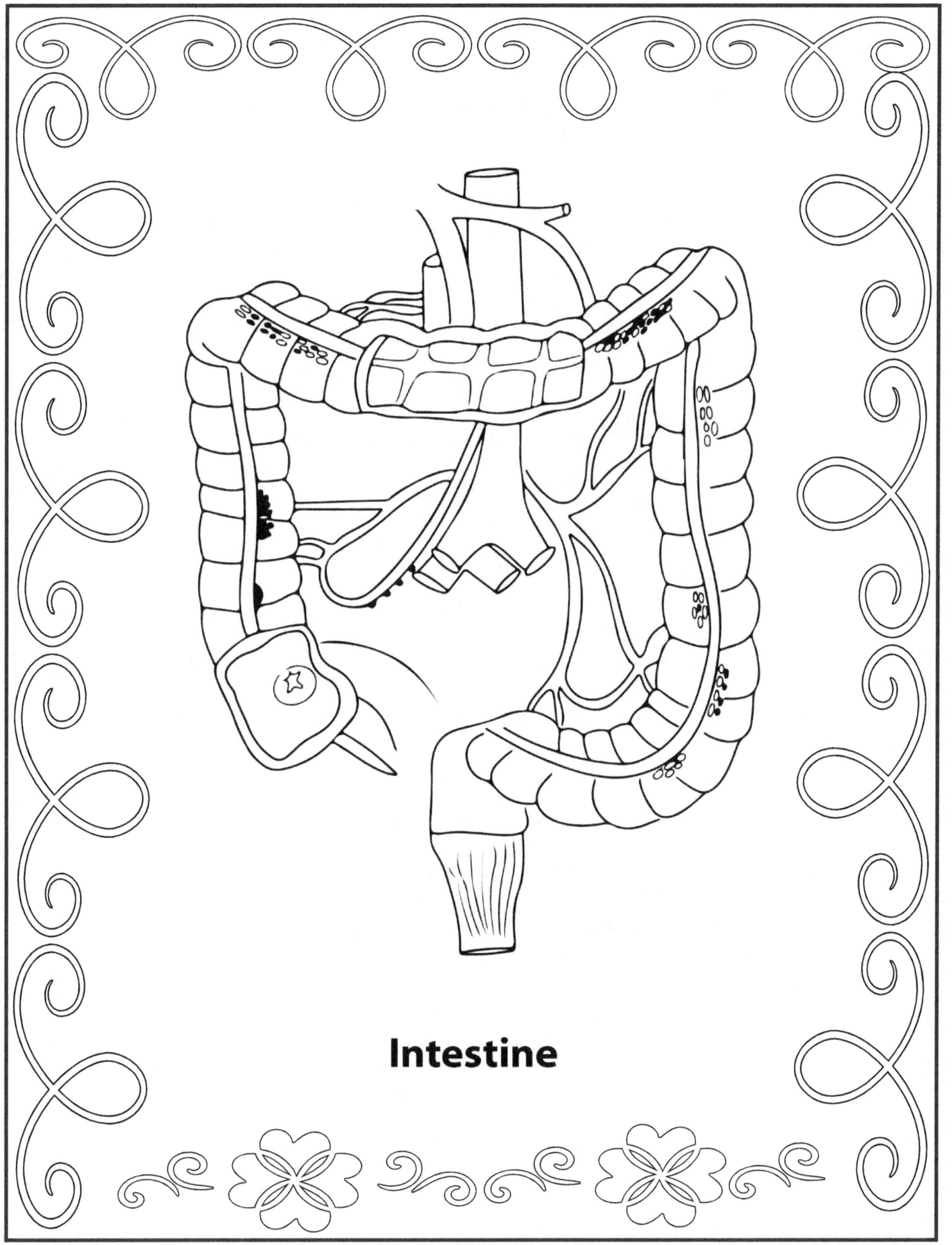

Intestine

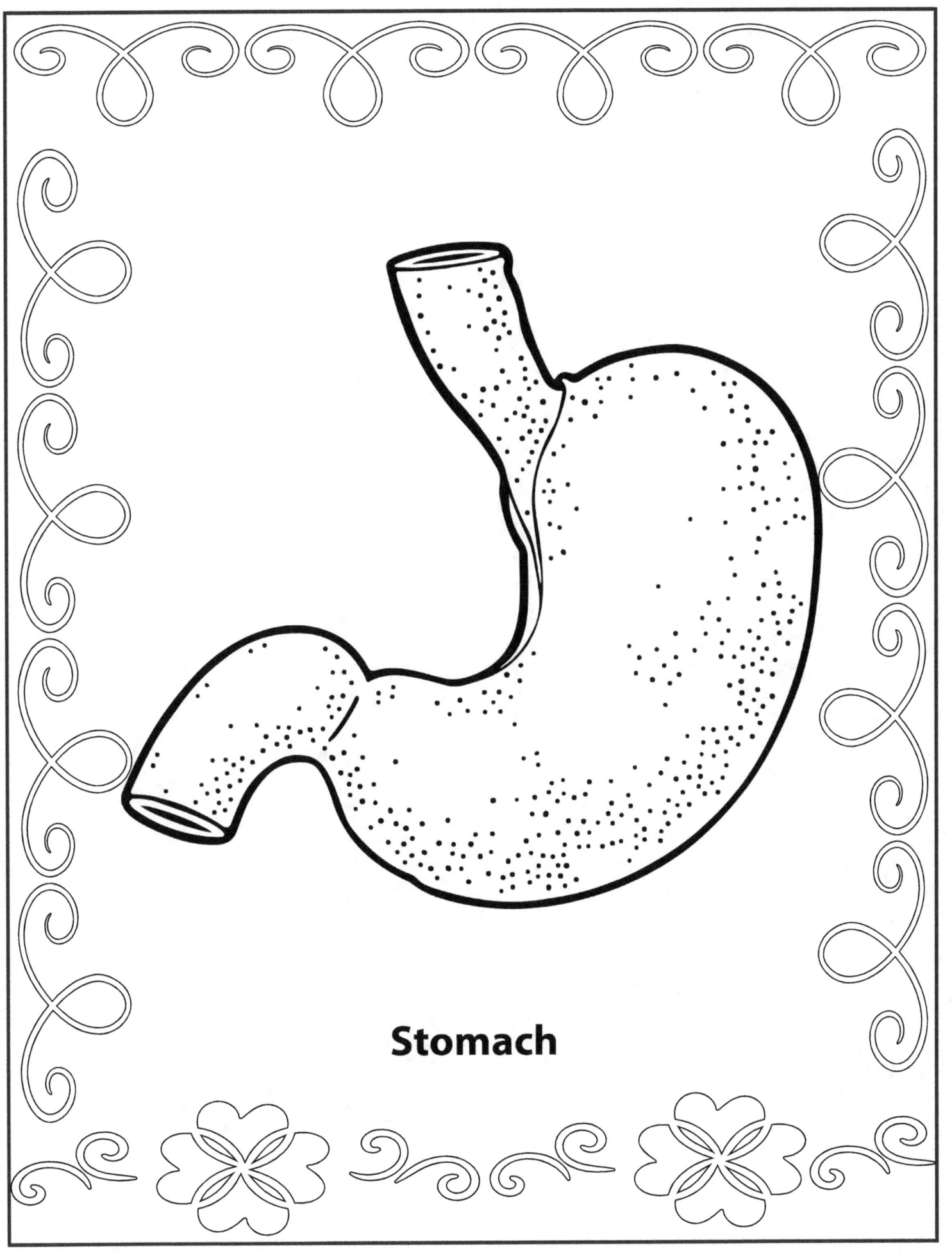
Stomach

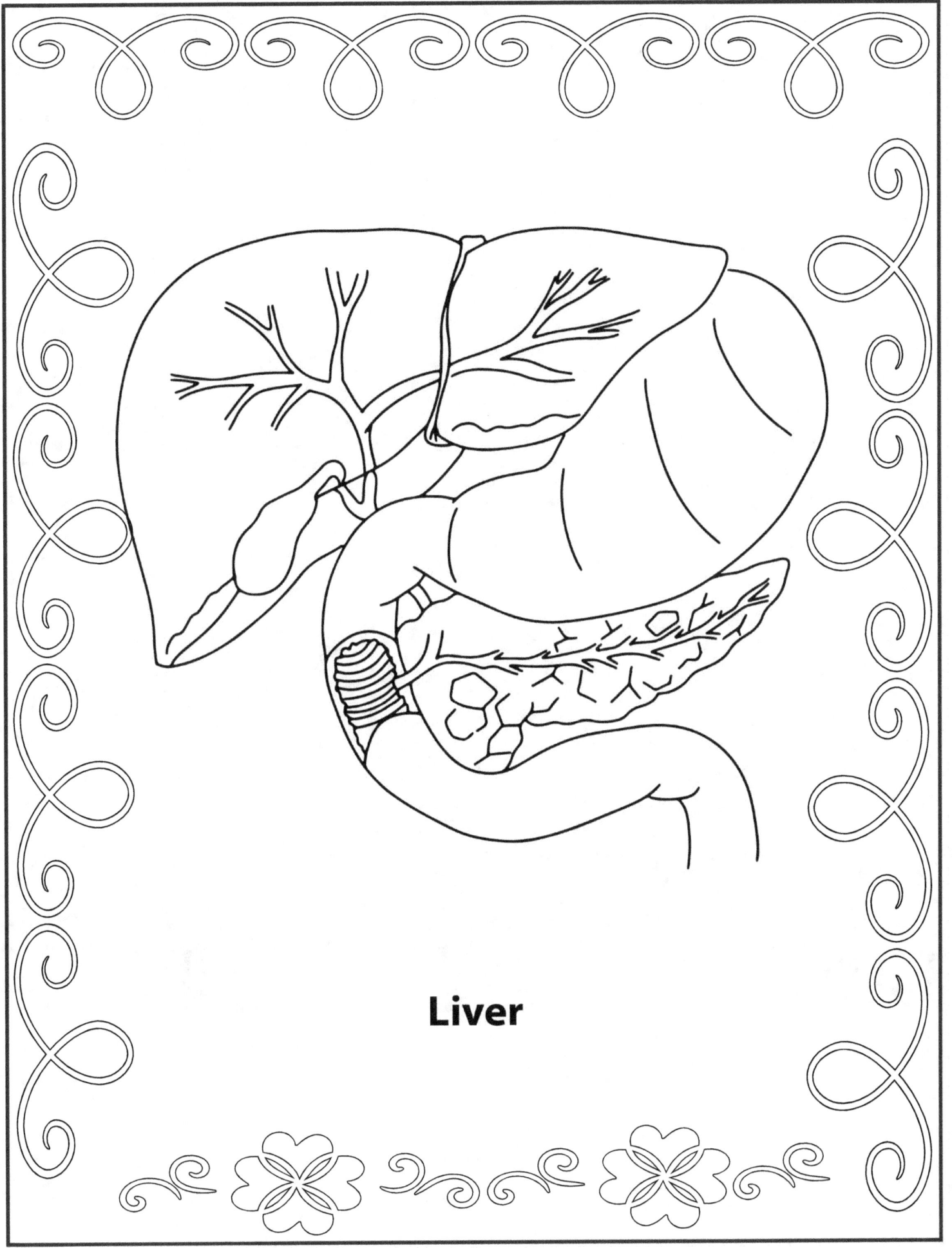
Liver

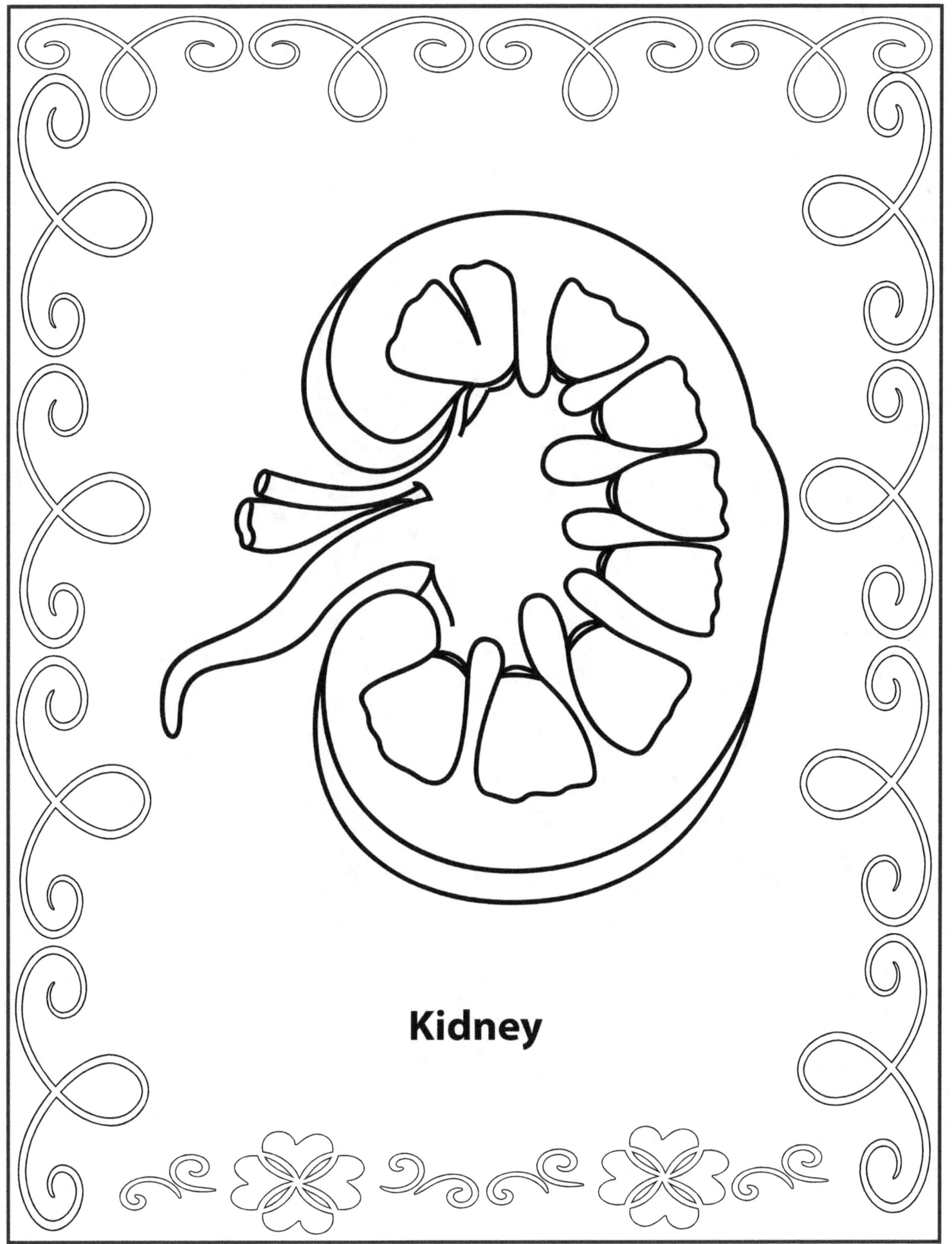

Kidney

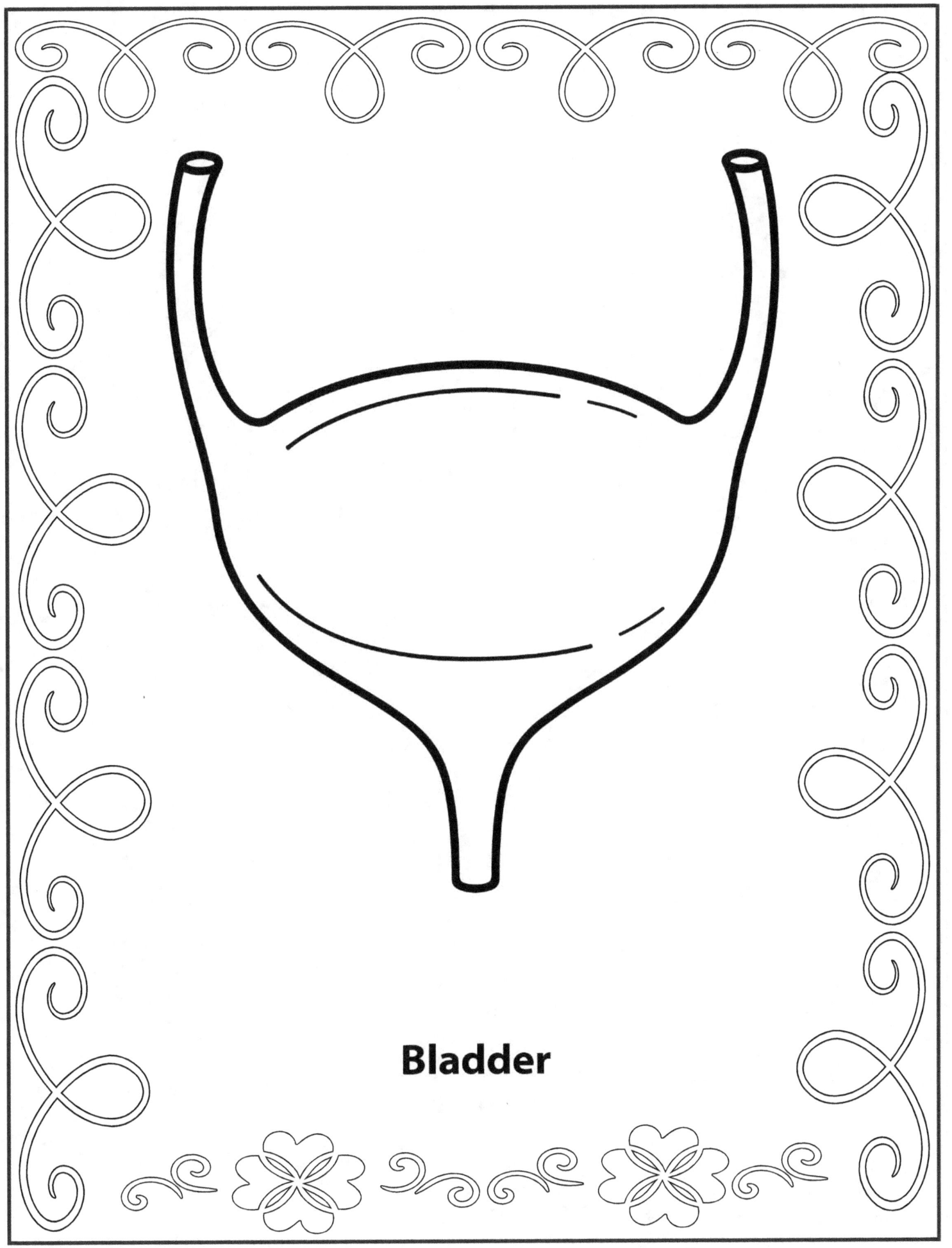

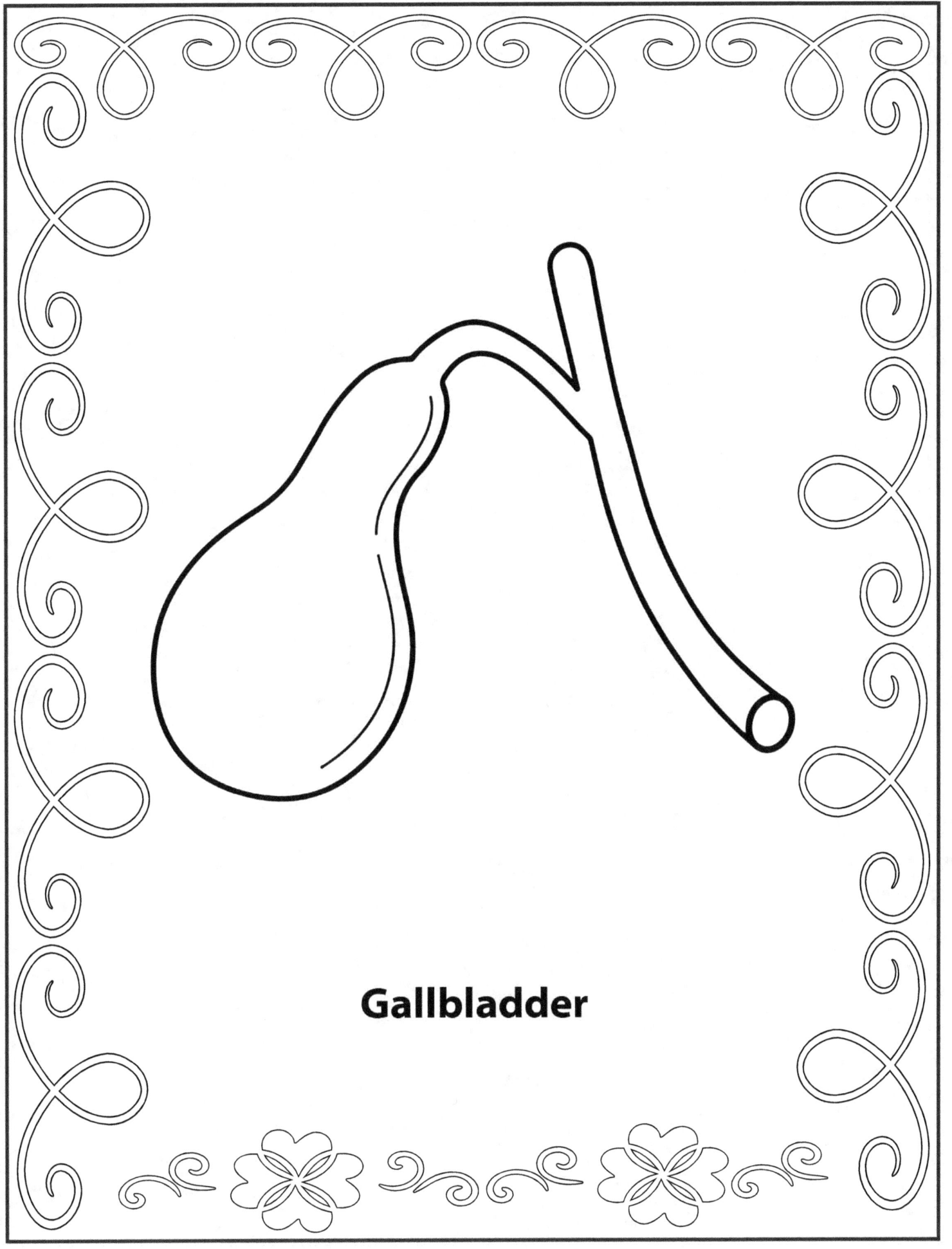

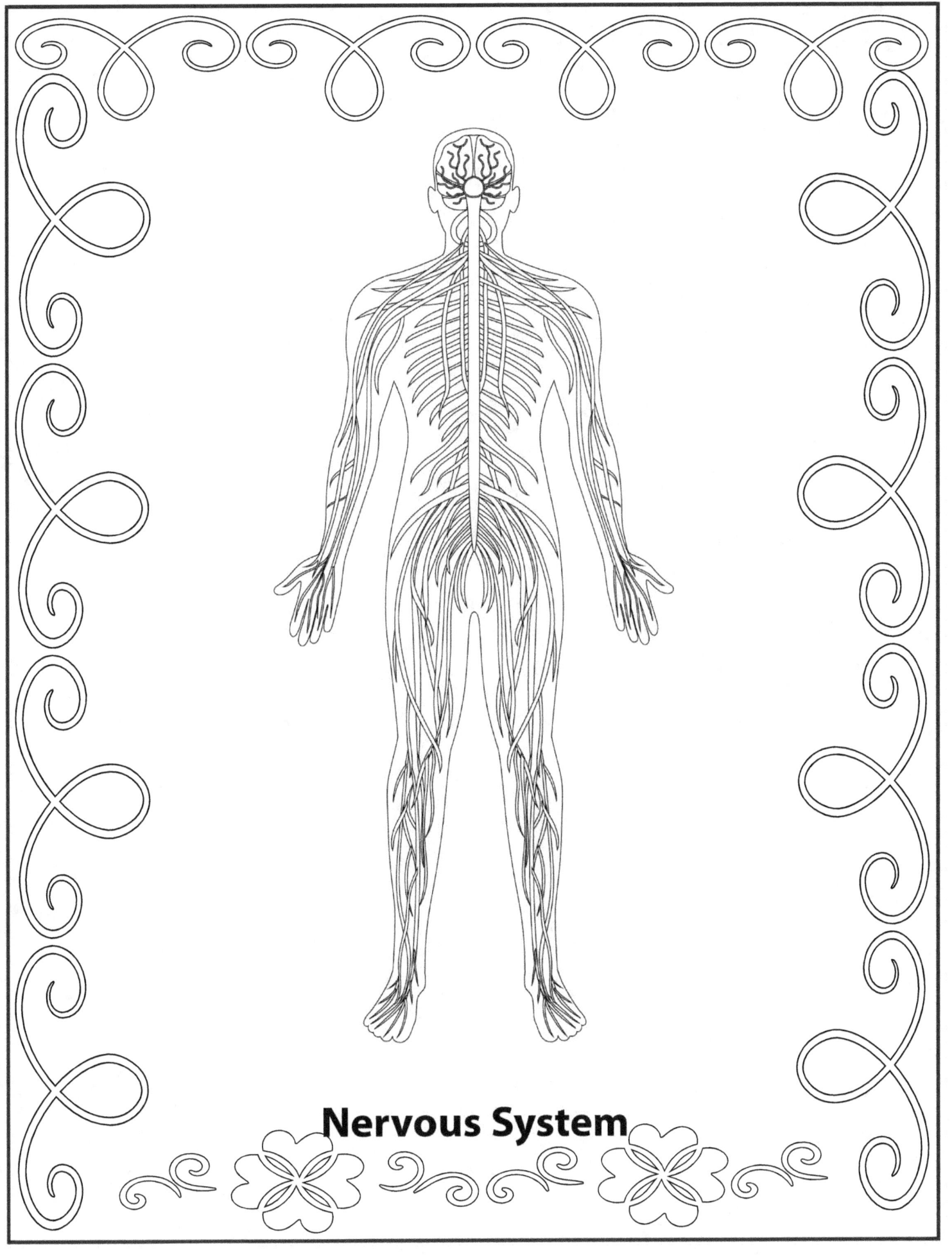

Nervous System

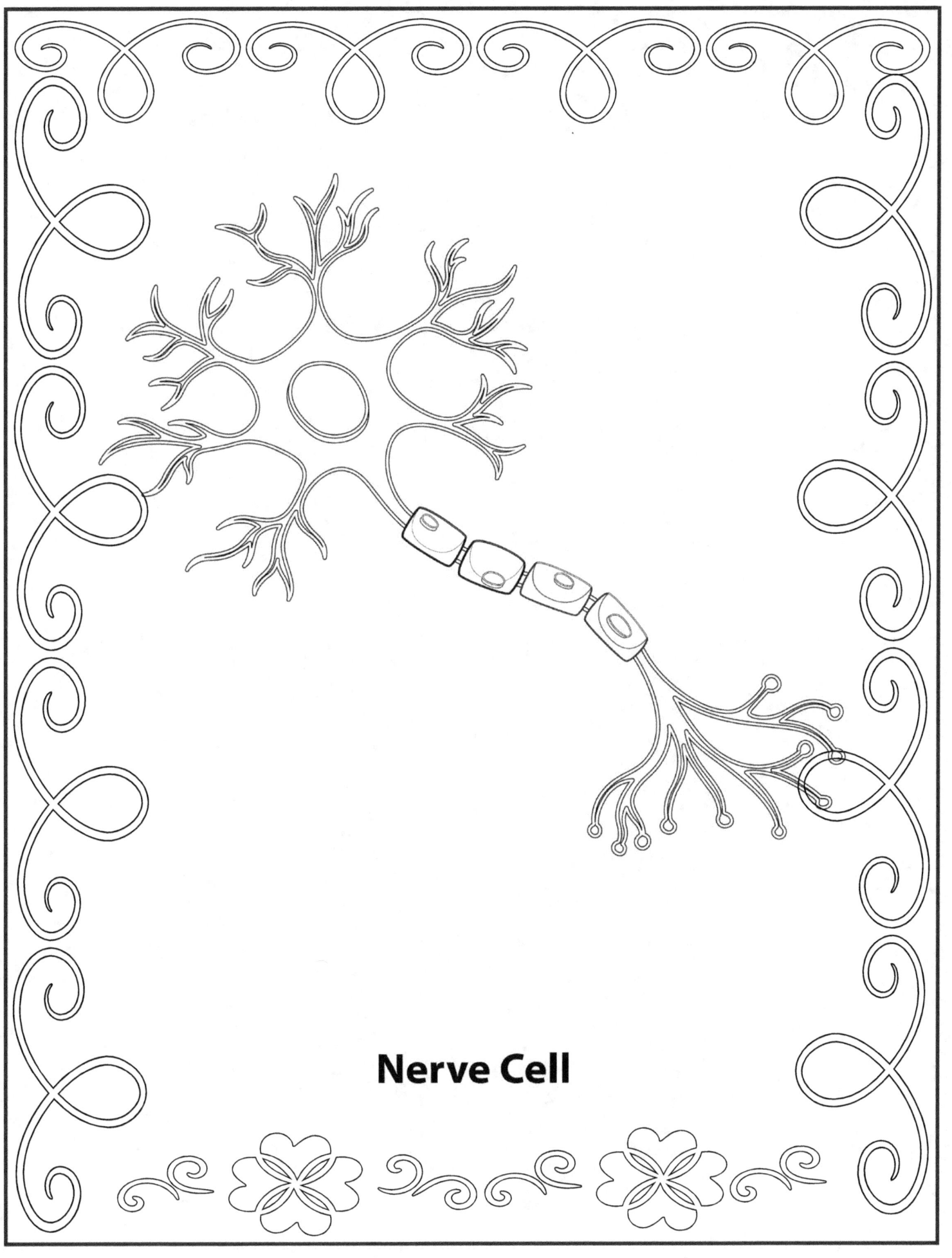

Nerve Cell

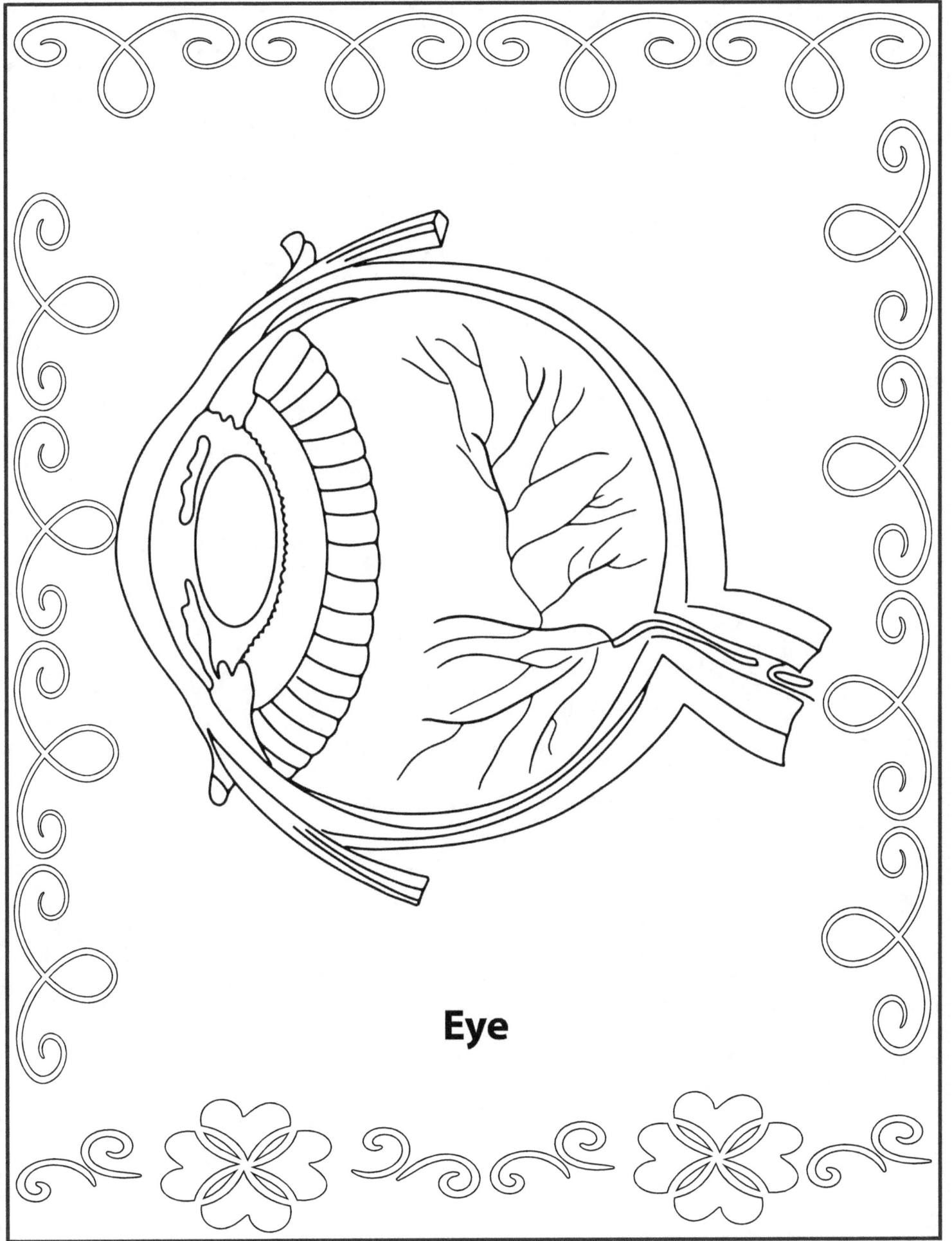

Eye

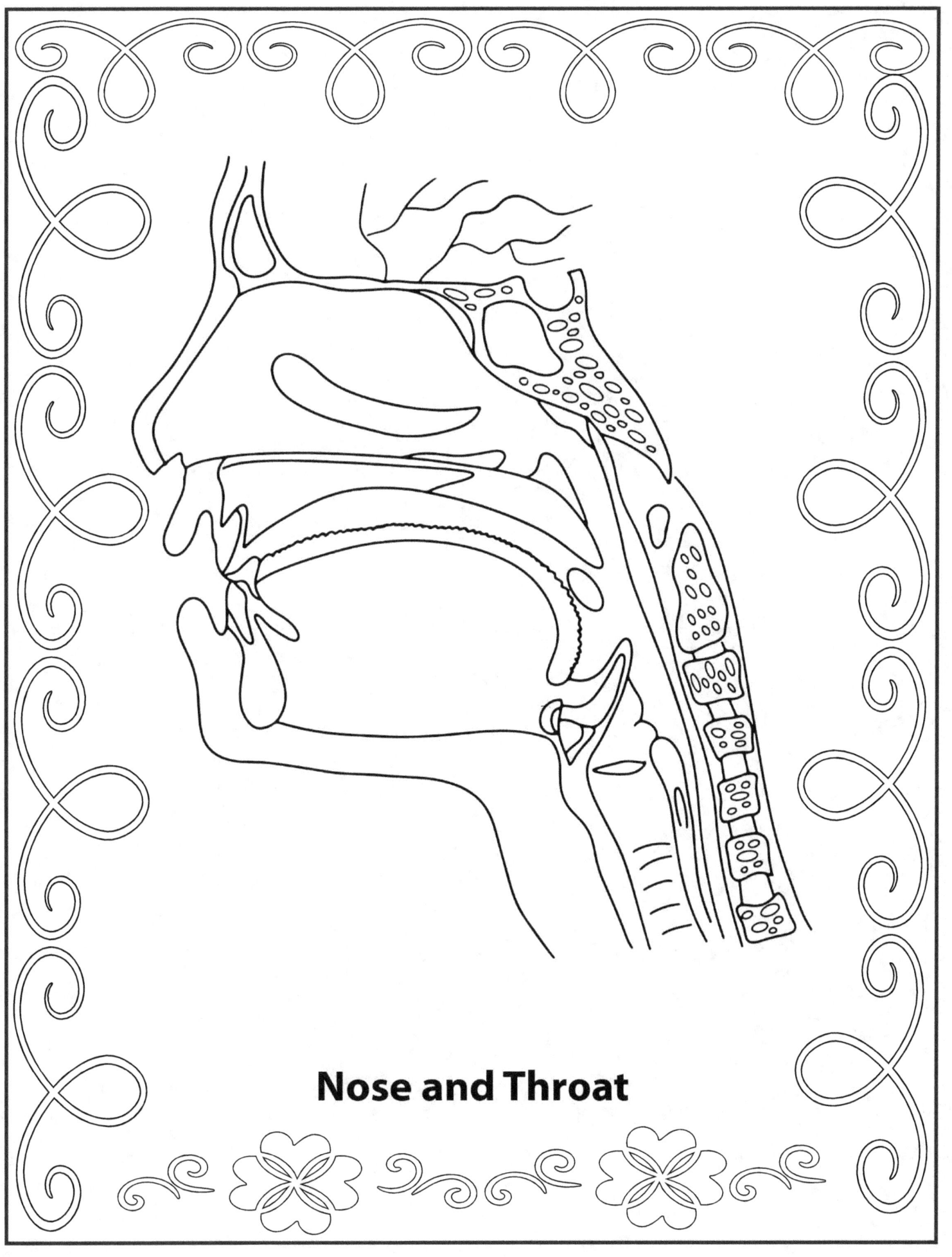

Nose and Throat

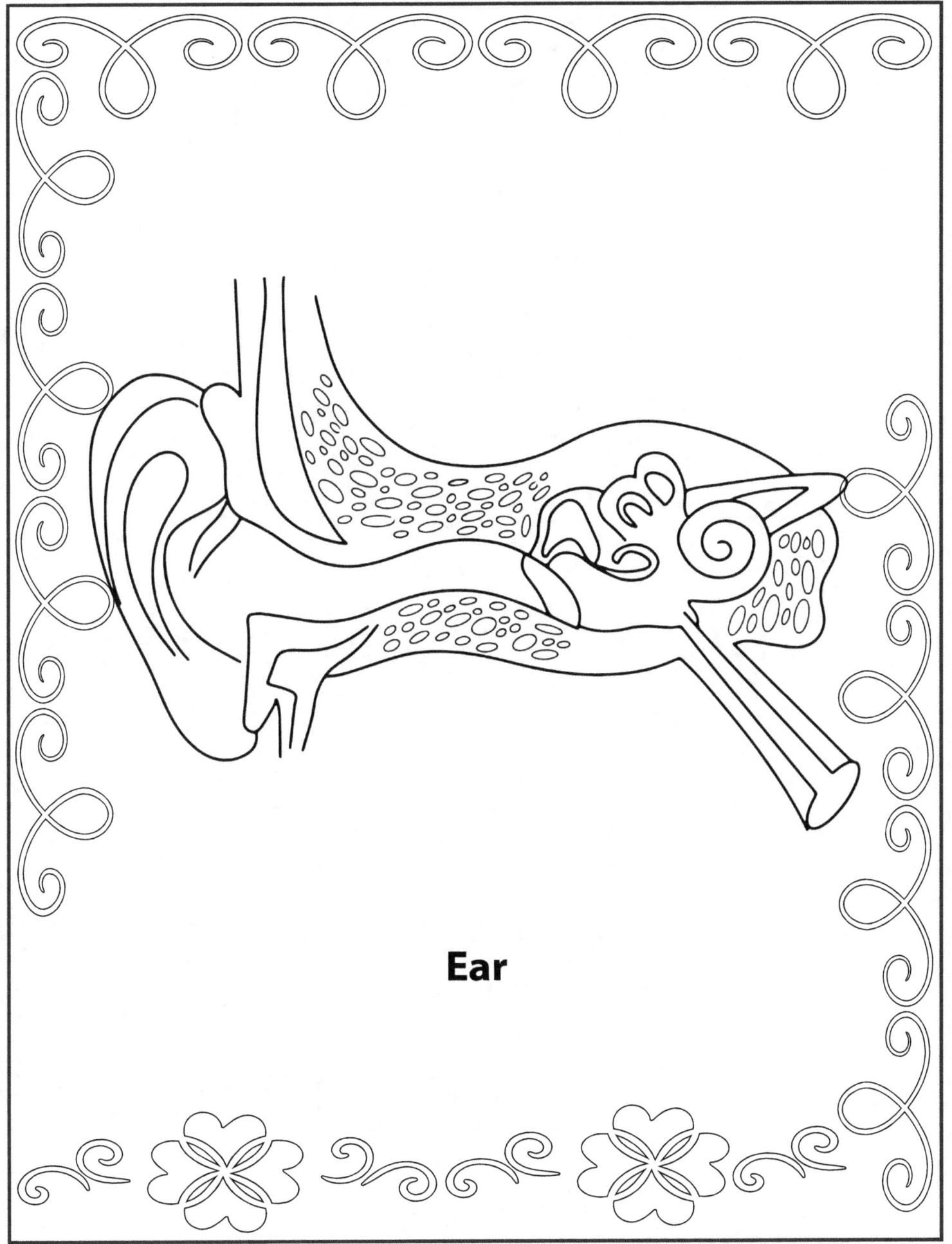

Ear

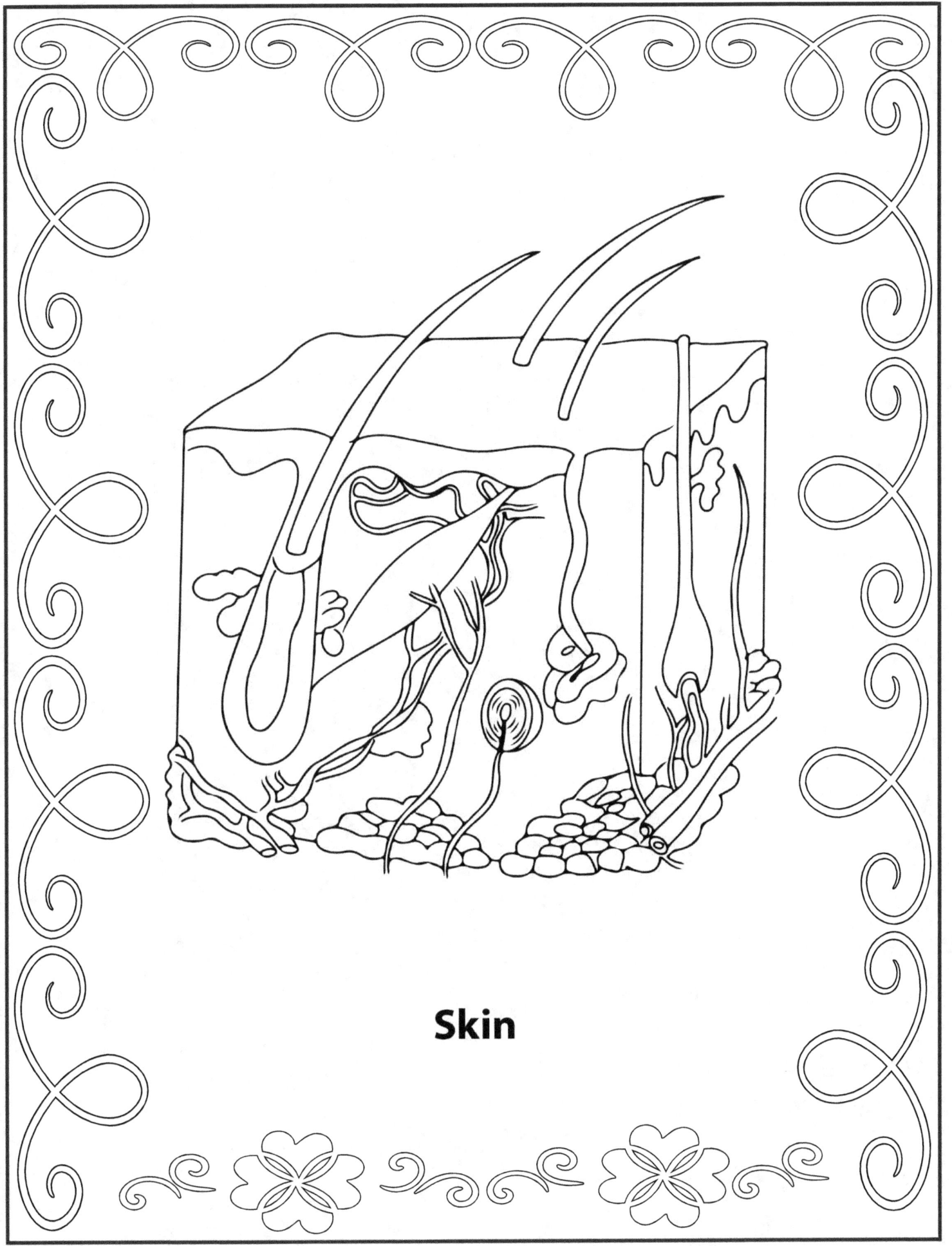

Skin

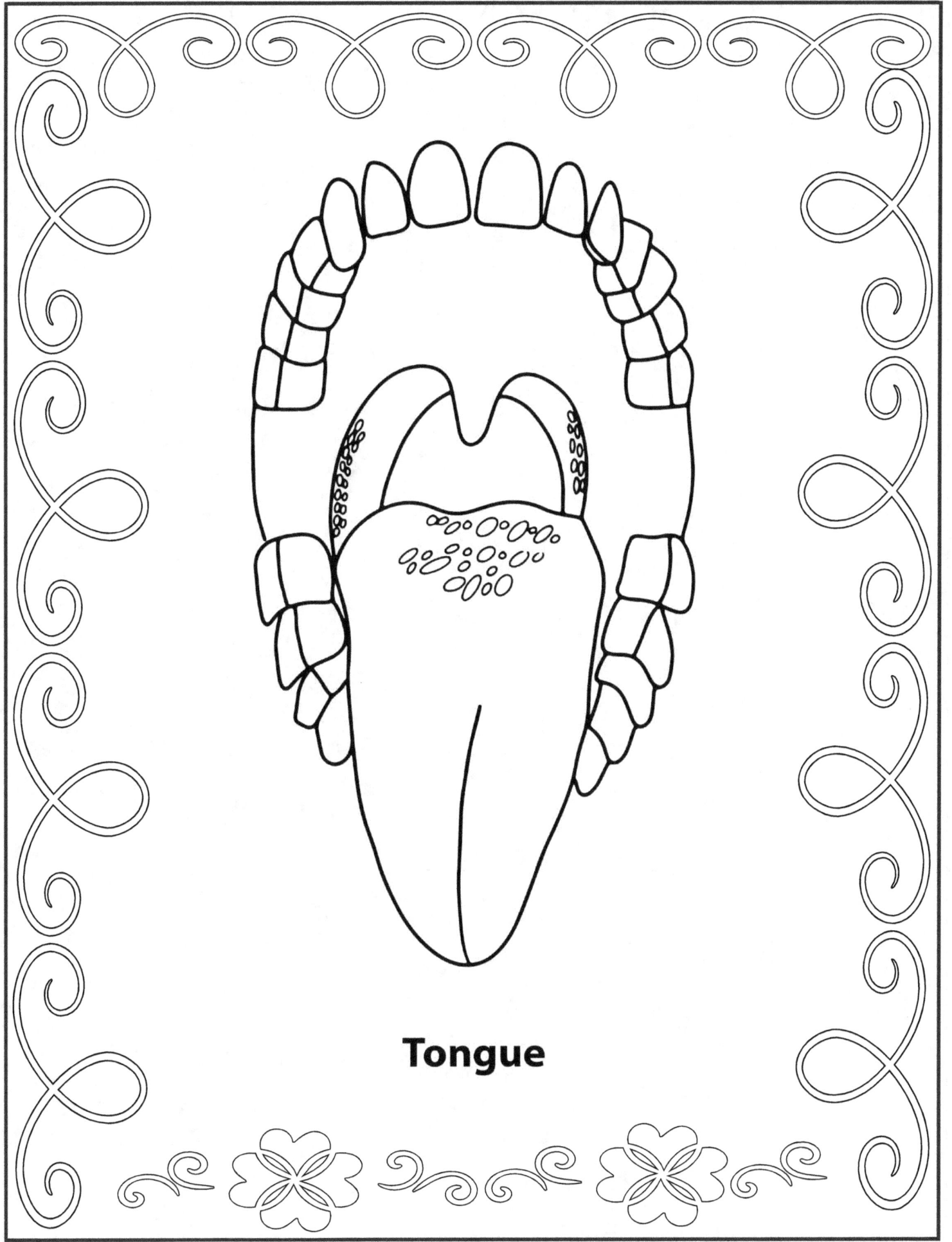
Tongue

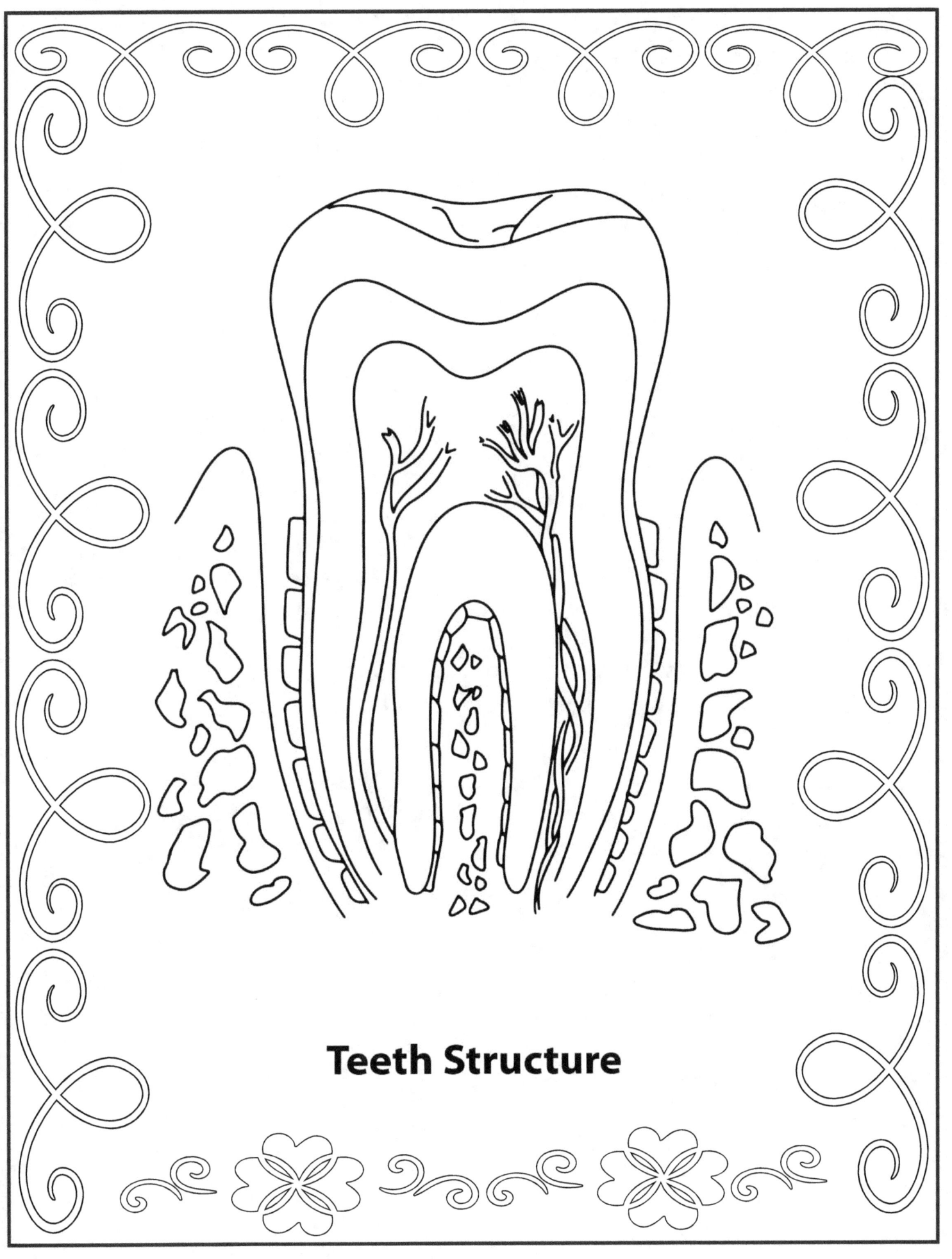

Teeth Structure

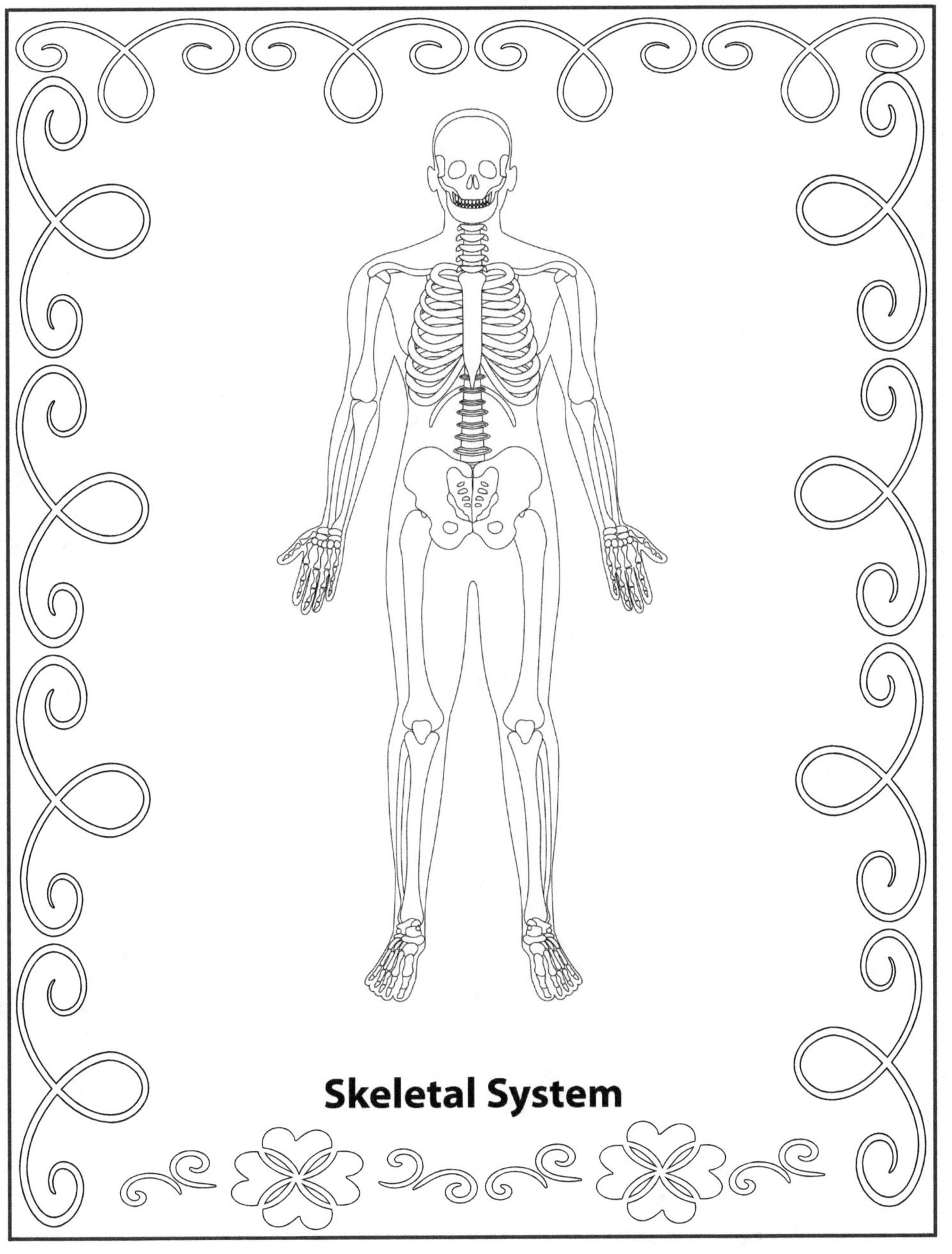

Skeletal System

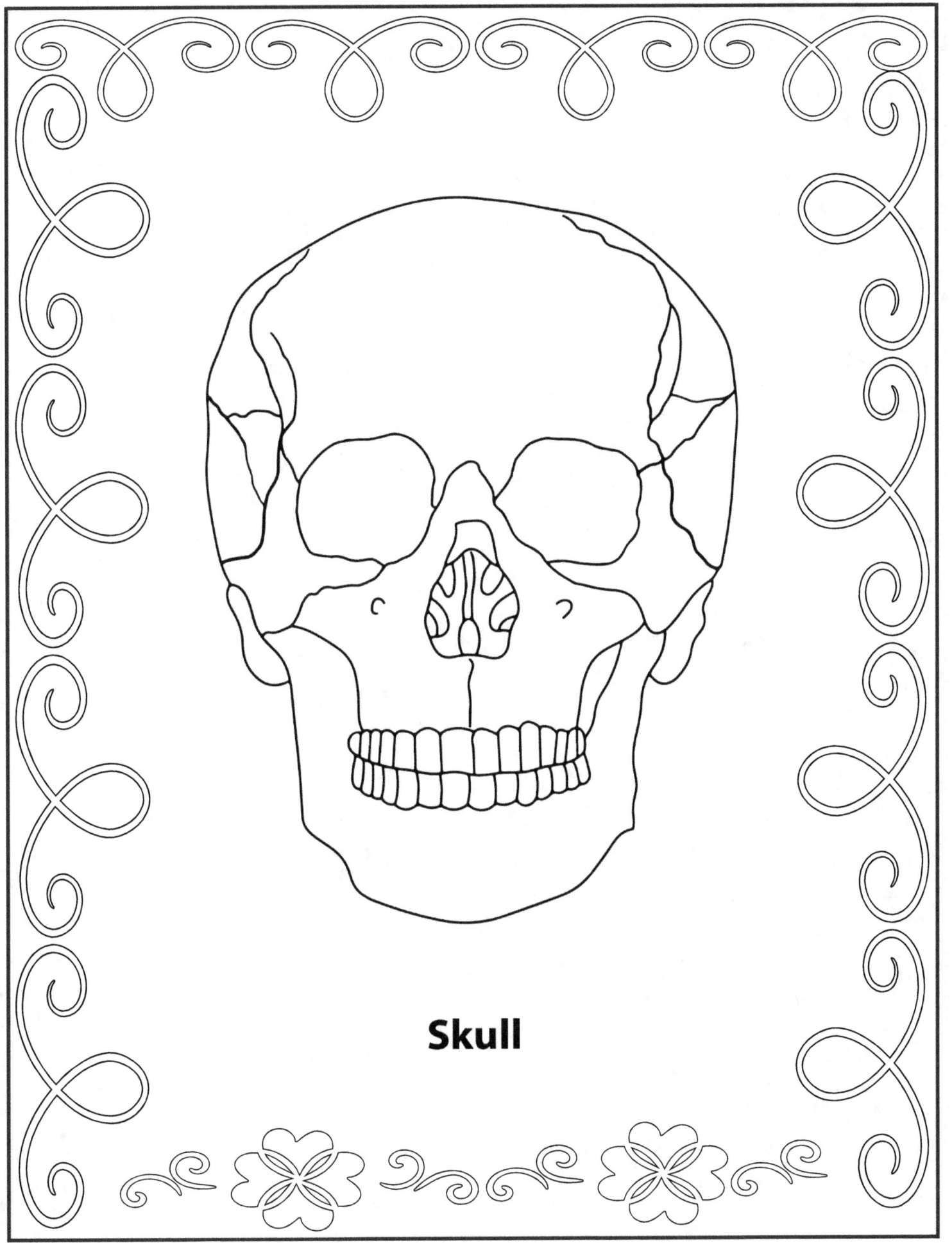

Skull

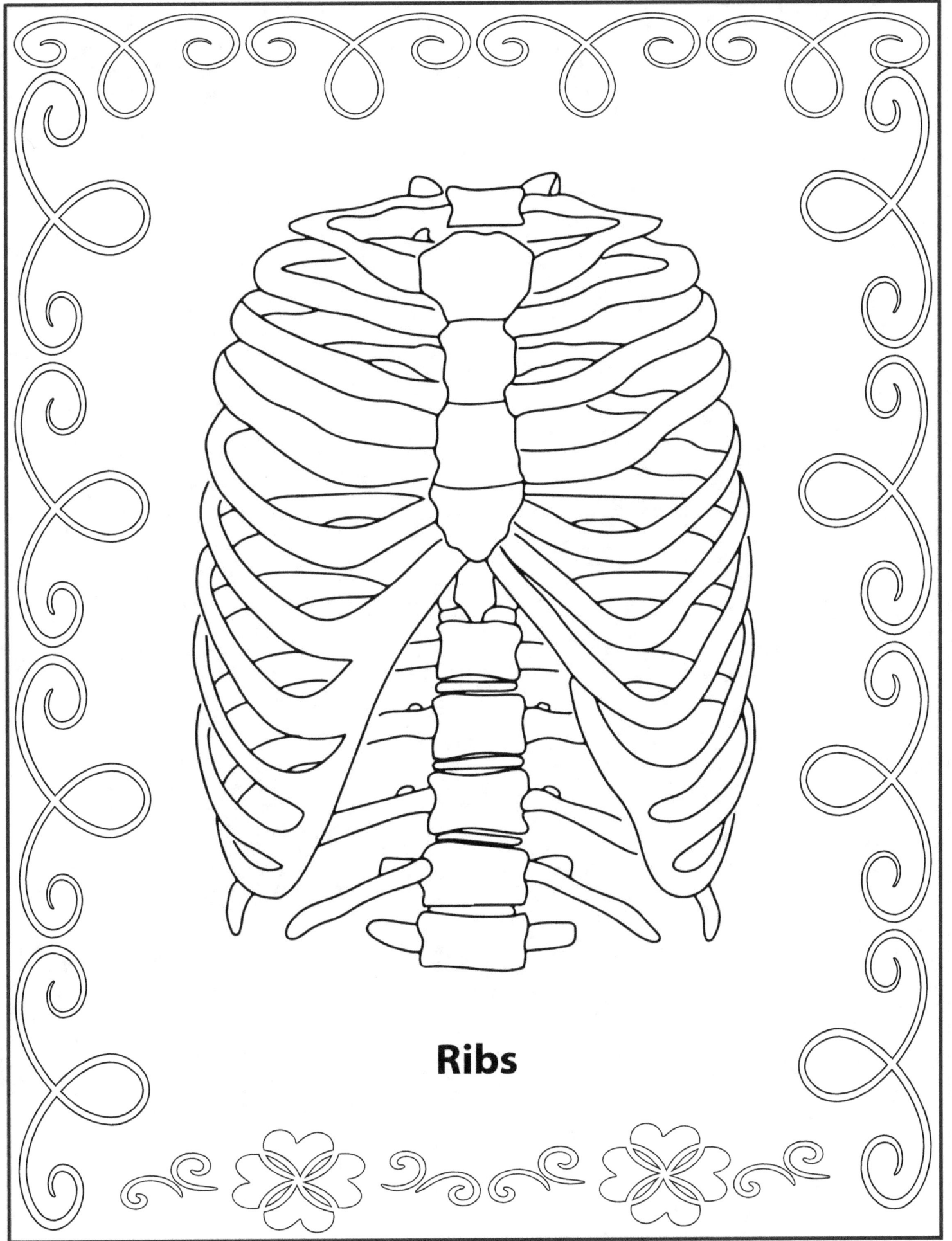
Ribs

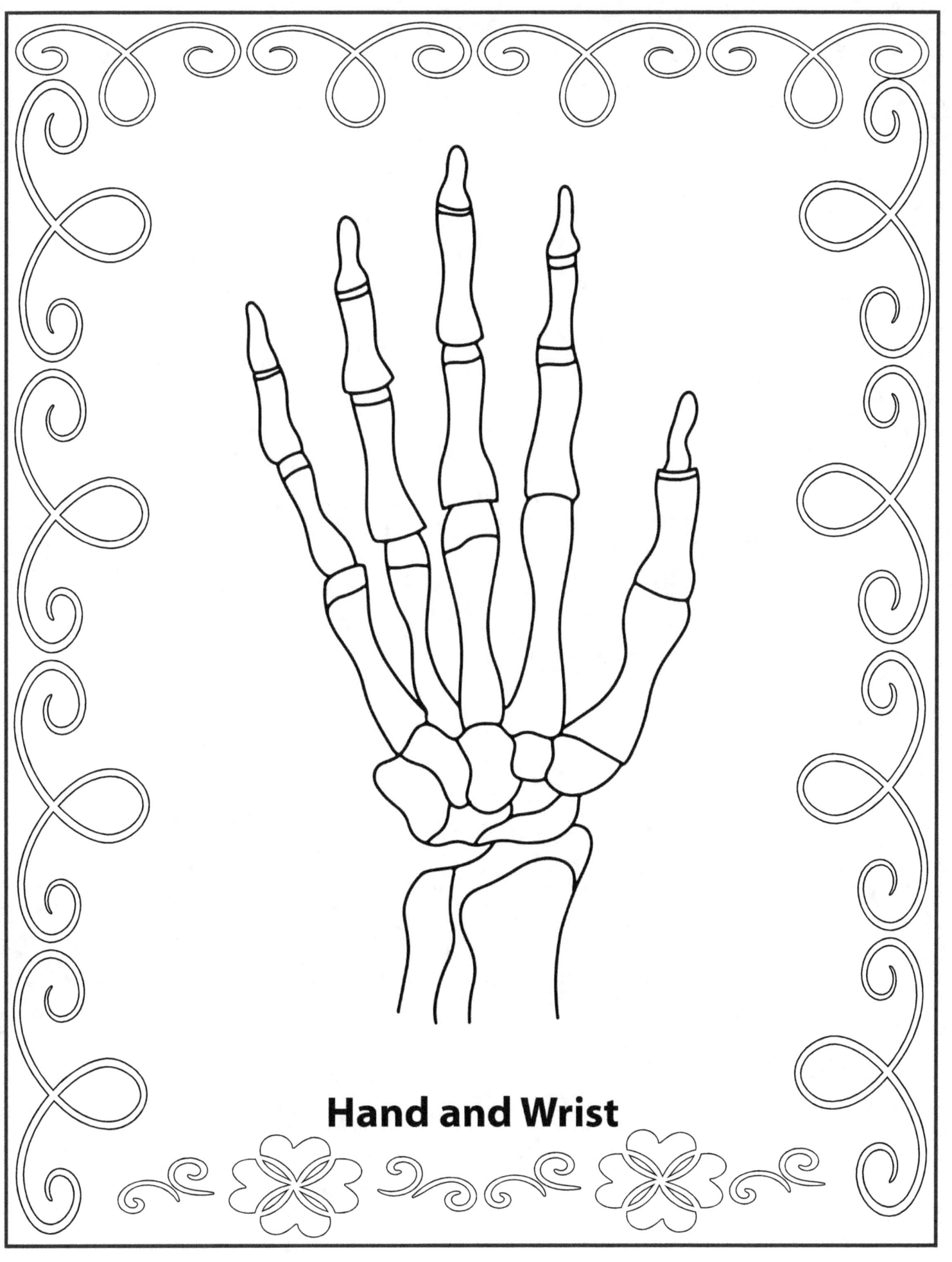

Hand and Wrist

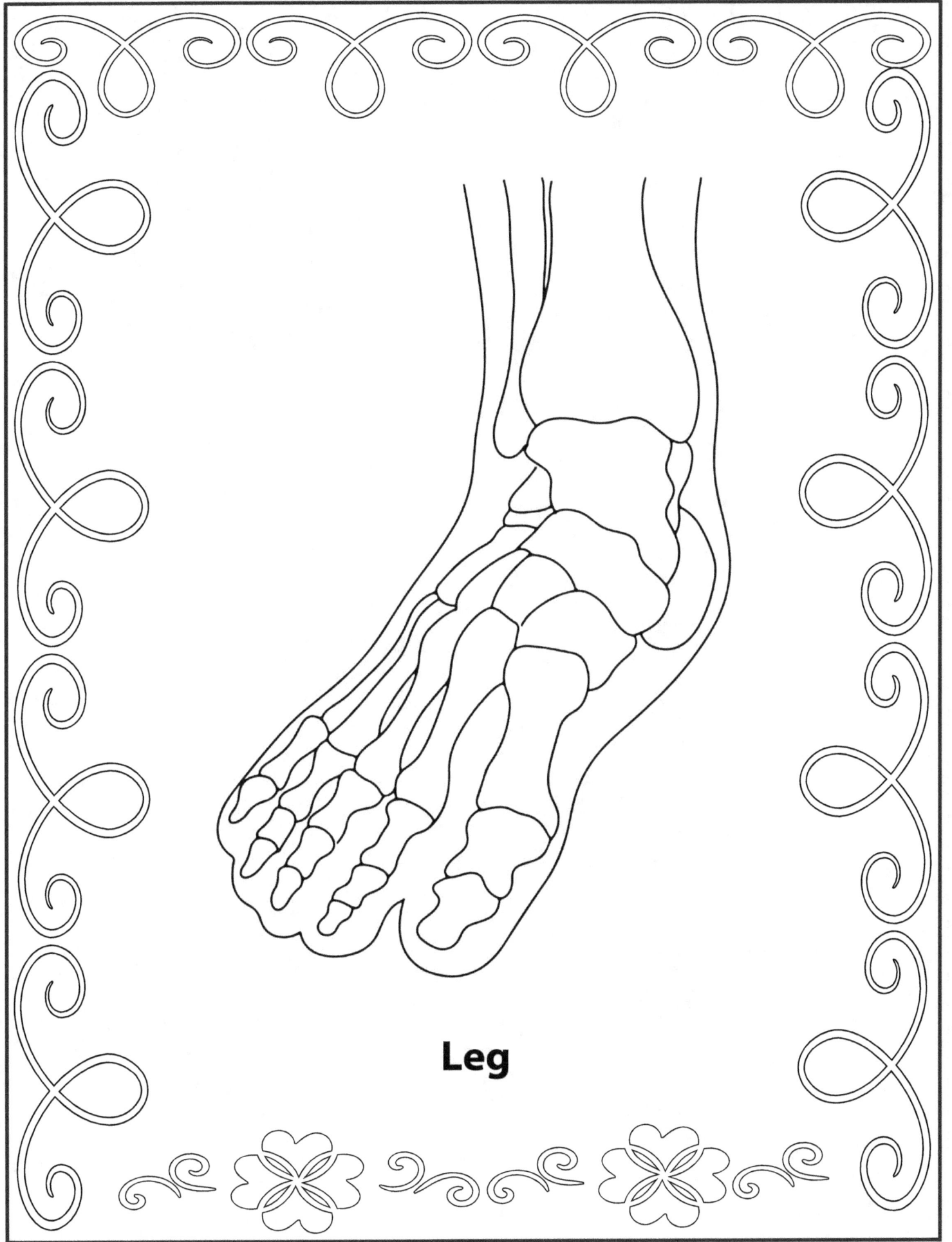

Leg

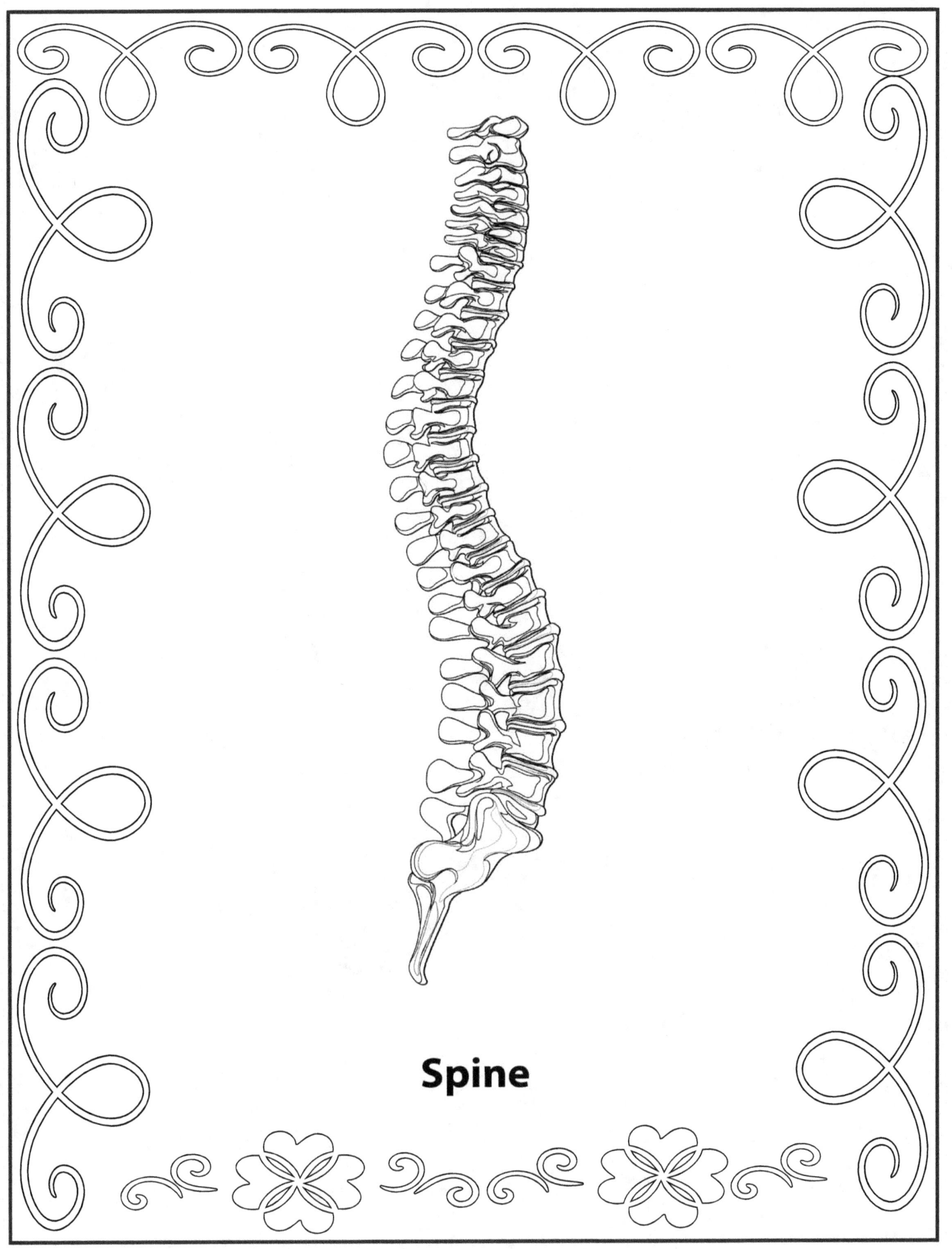

Spine

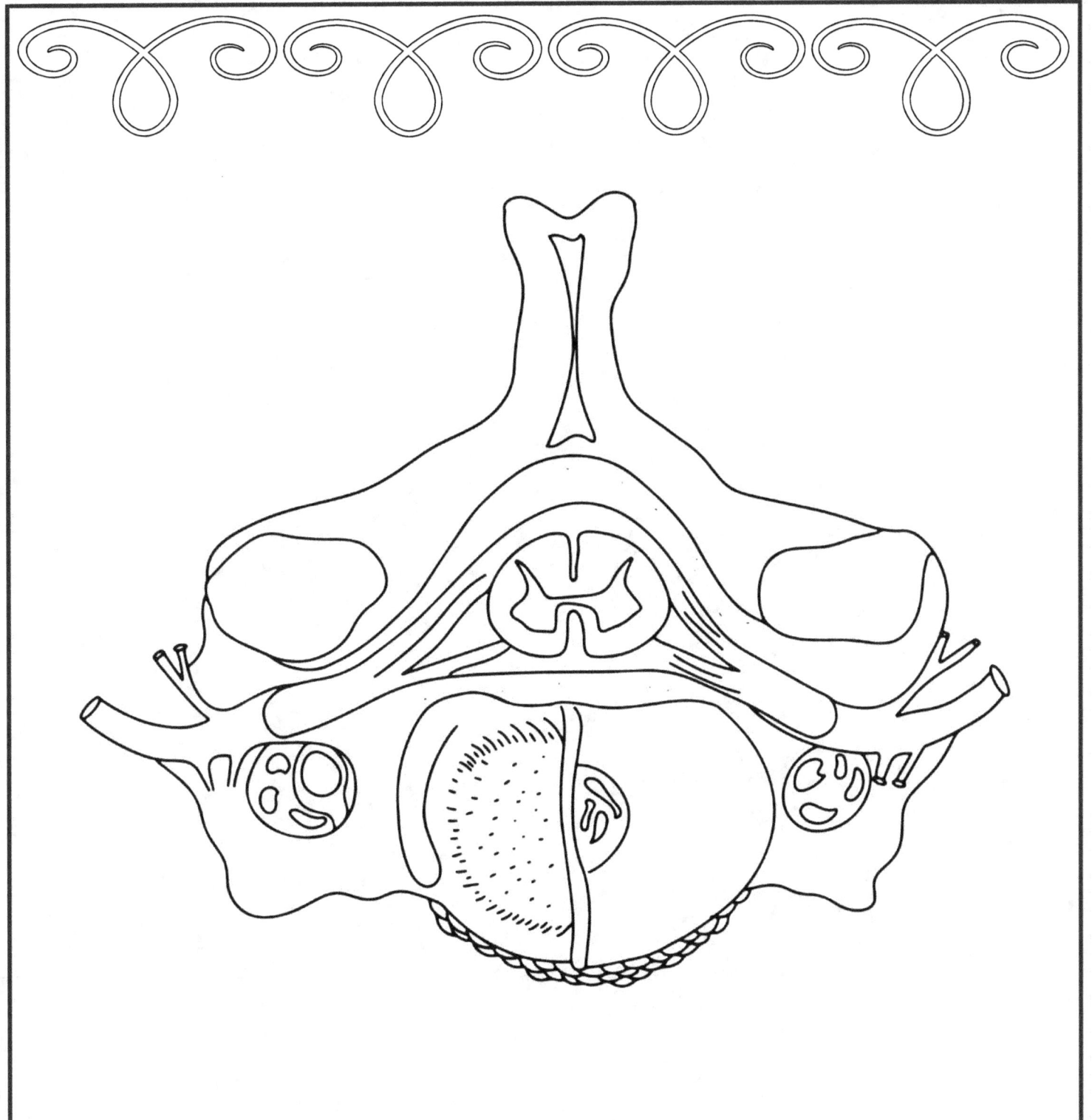

Spinal Cord

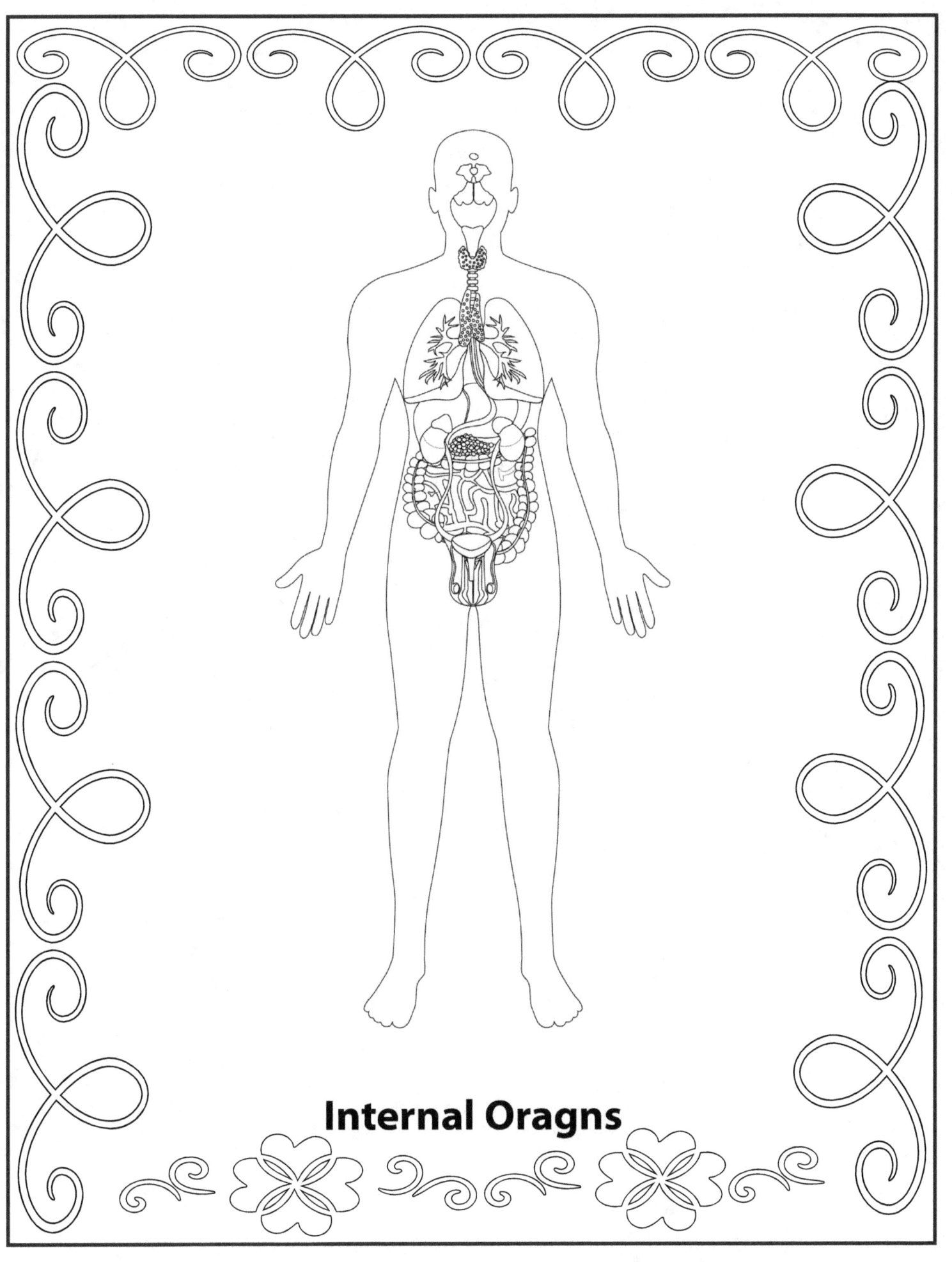

Internal Oragns

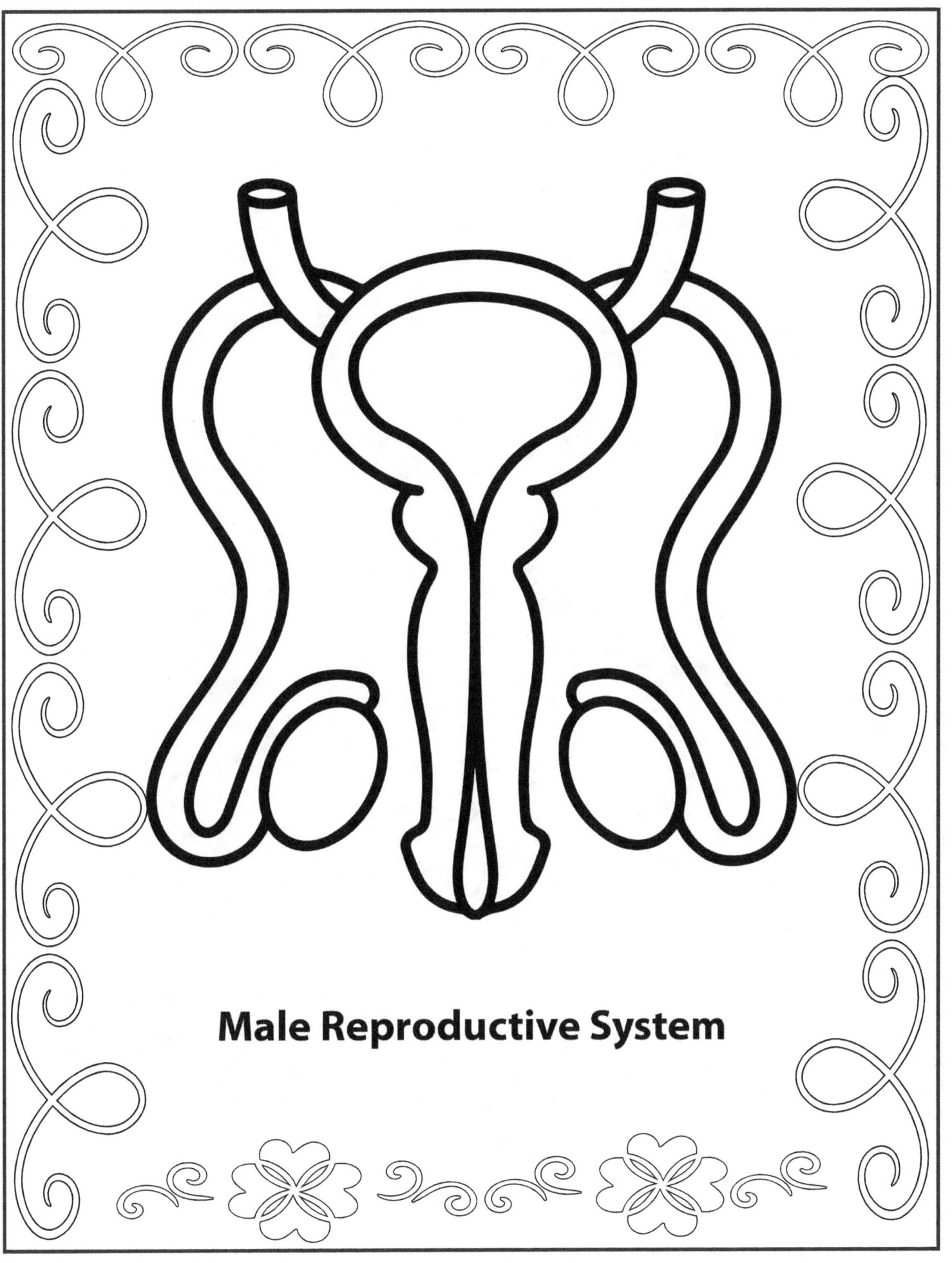

Male Reproductive System

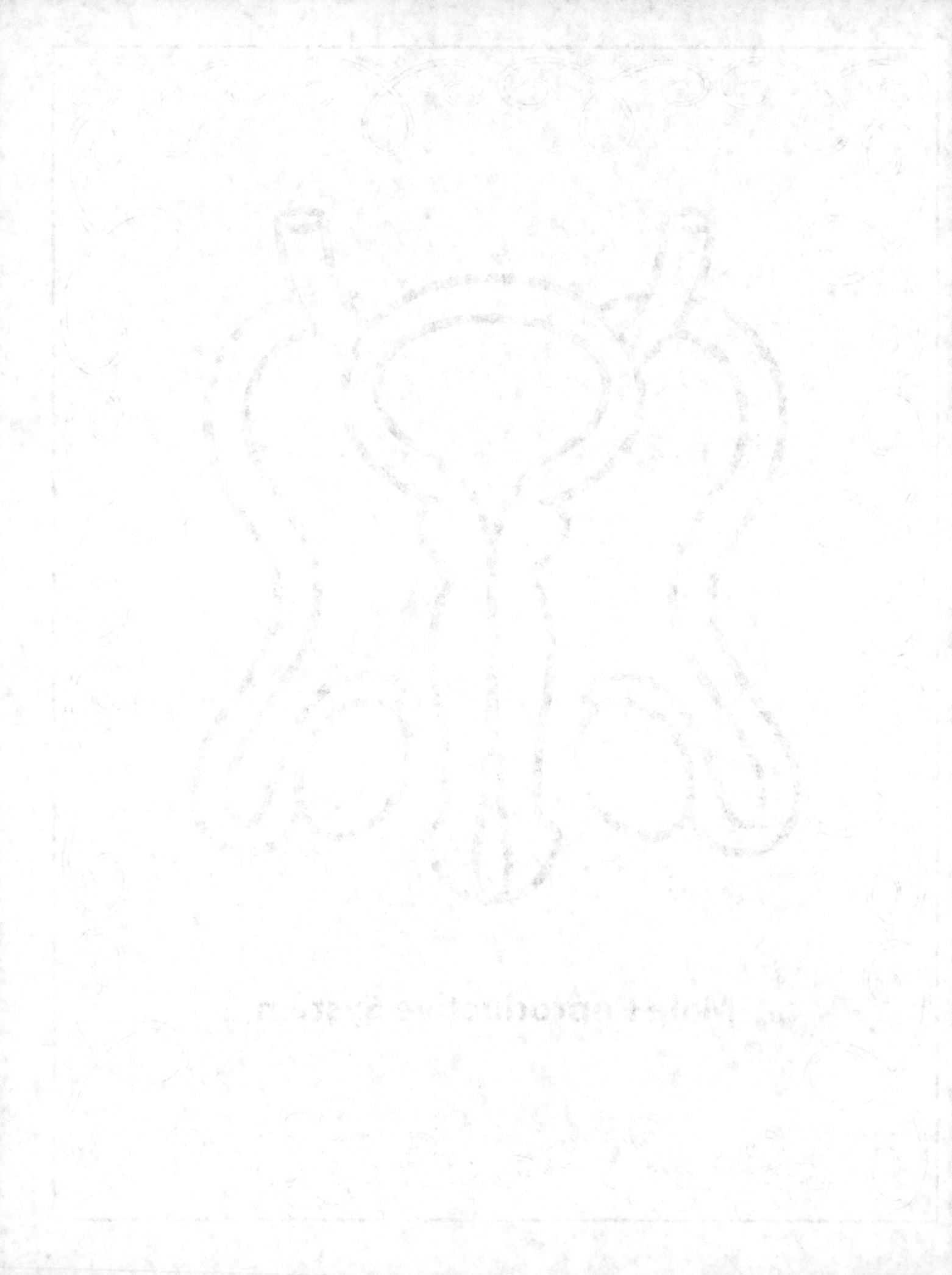

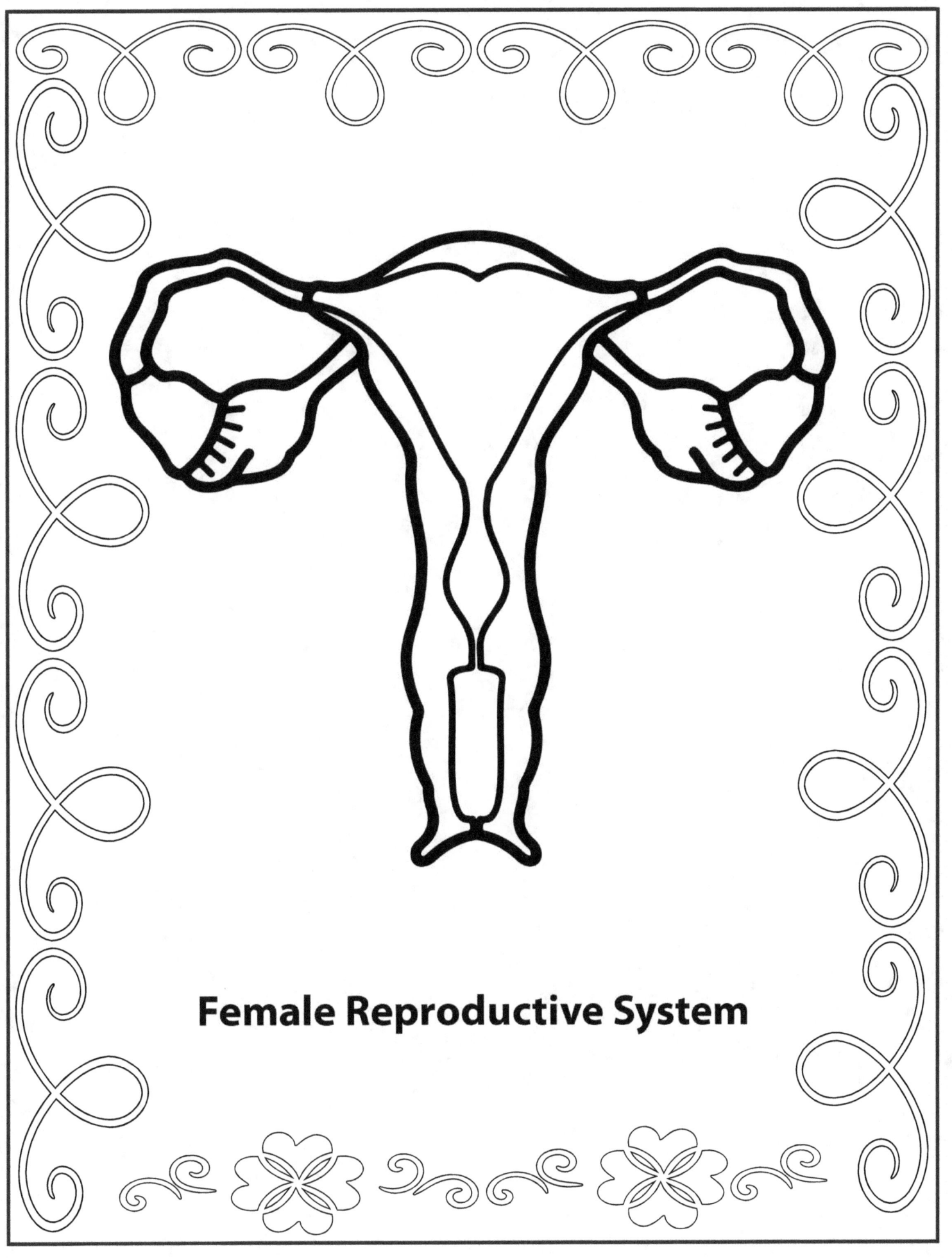

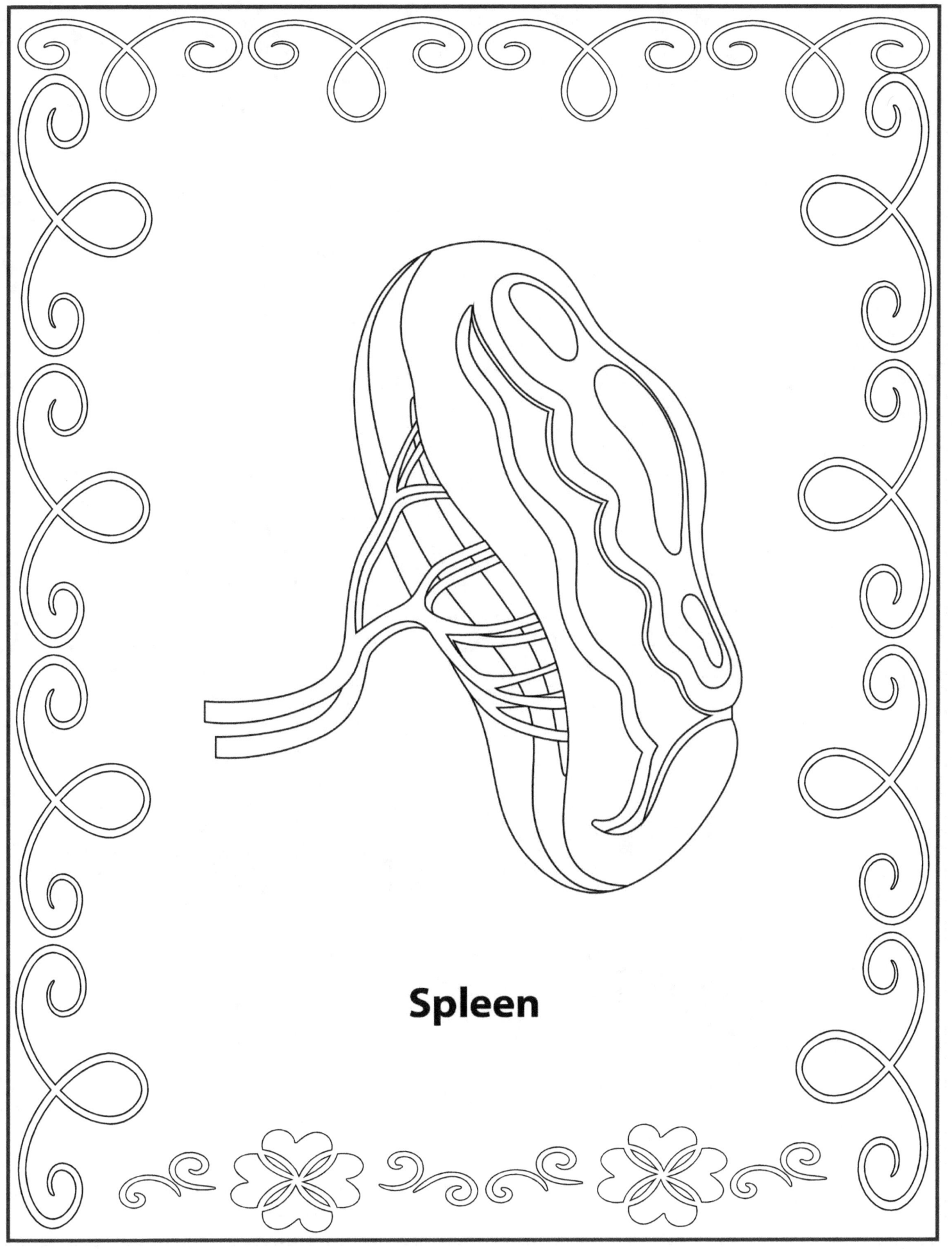

Spleen

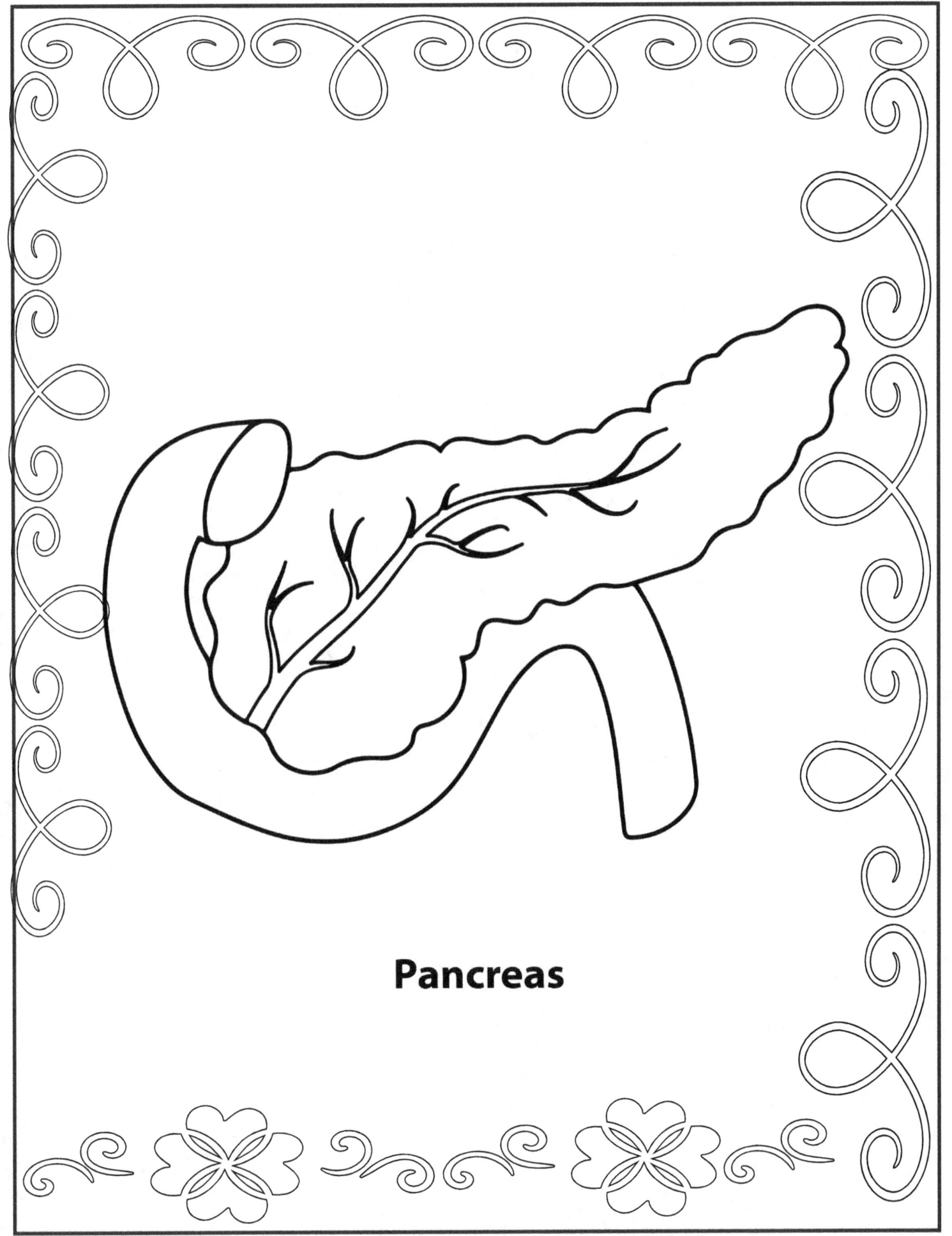

Pancreas

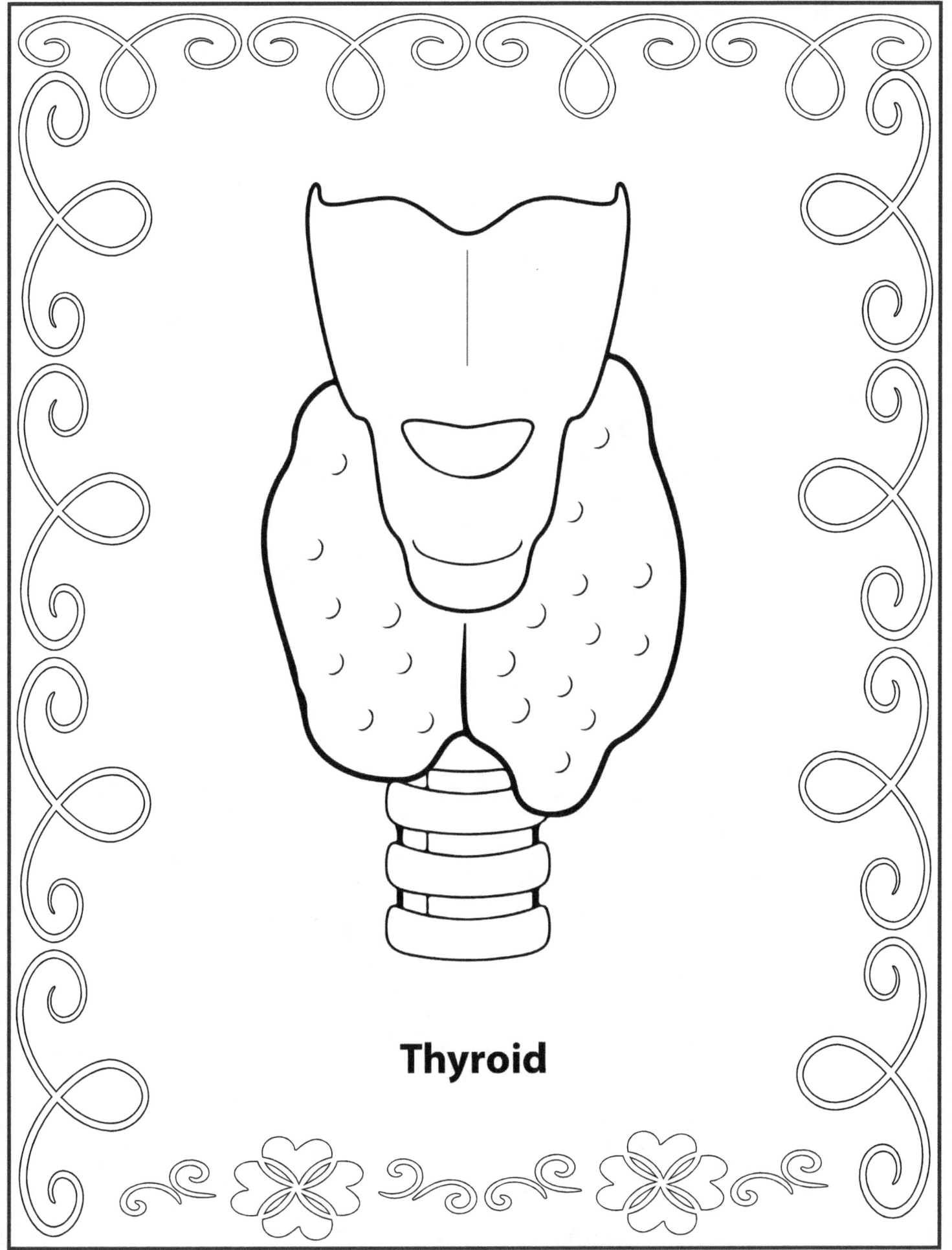
Thyroid

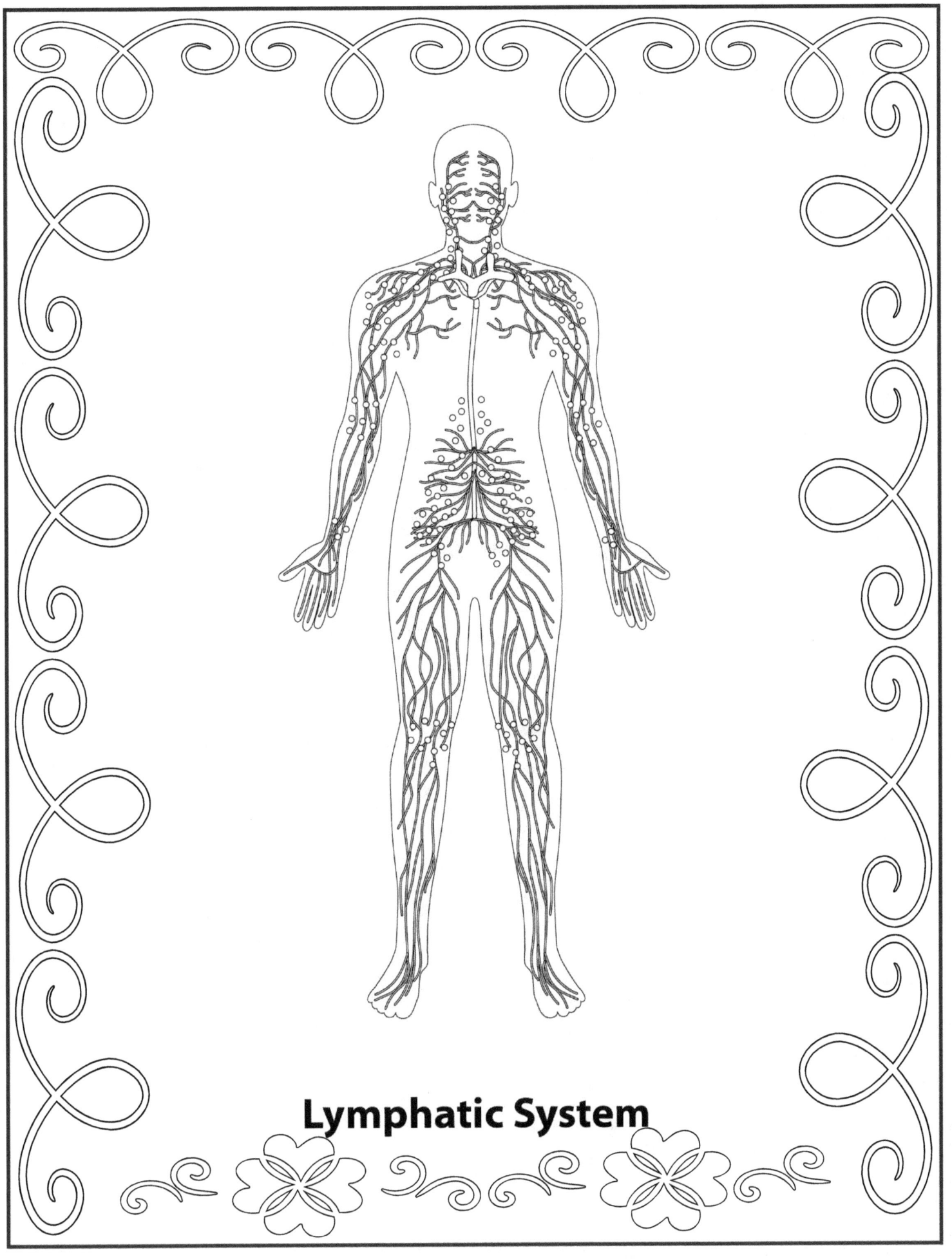

Lymphatic System

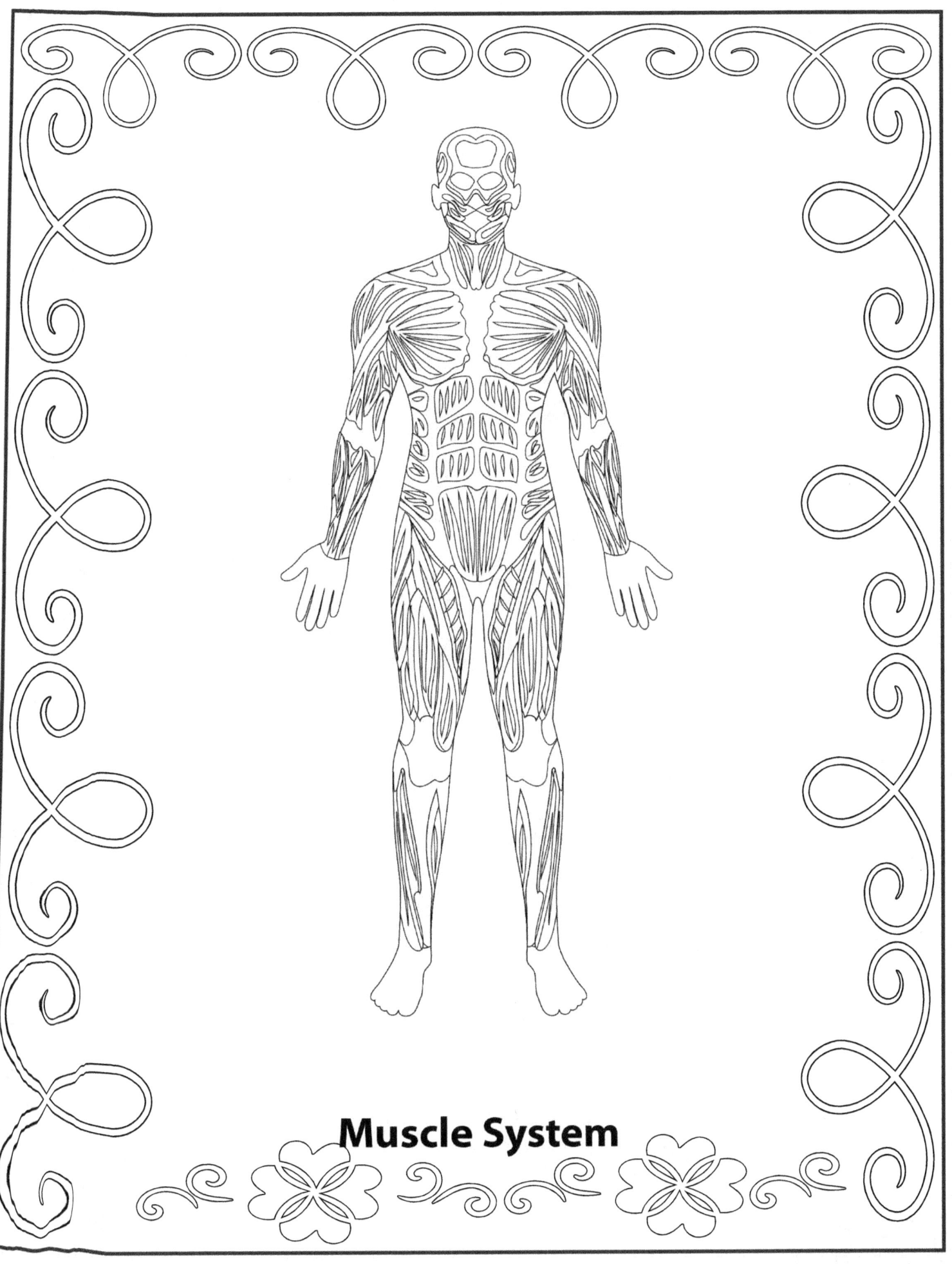